O A P L
OXFORD AMERICAN PSYCHIATRY LIBRARY

Bipolar Disorder

D0814945

O A P L
OXFORD AMERICAN PSYCHIATRY LIBRARY

Bipolar Disorder

Stephen M. Strakowski, MD

Senior Vice President for Strategic Planning & Business
Development, UC Health
The Dr. Stanley and Mickey Kaplan Professor and Chairman
Department of Psychiatry & Behavioral Neuroscience
University of Cincinnati College of Medicine
Cincinnati, OH

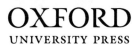

OXFORD
UNIVERSITY PRESS

OXFORD
UNIVERSITY PRESS

Oxford University Press is a department of the University of
Oxford. It furthers the University's objective of excellence in research,
scholarship, and education by publishing worldwide.

Oxford   New York
Auckland   Cape Town   Dar es Salaam   Hong Kong   Karachi
Kuala Lumpur   Madrid   Melbourne   Mexico City   Nairobi
New Delhi   Shanghai   Taipei   Toronto

With offices in
Argentina   Austria   Brazil   Chile   Czech Republic   France   Greece
Guatemala   Hungary   Italy   Japan   Poland   Portugal   Singapore
South Korea   Switzerland   Thailand   Turkey   Ukraine   Vietnam

Oxford is a registered trademark of Oxford University Press
in the UK and certain other countries.

Published in the United States of America by
Oxford University Press
198 Madison Avenue, New York, NY 10016

© Oxford University Press 2014

Library of Congress Cataloging-in-Publication Data
Strakowski, Stephen M., author.
Bipolar disorder / Stephen M. Strakowski.
    p. ; cm.—(Oxford American psychiatry library)
Includes bibliographical references.
ISBN 978-0-19-999568-4 (alk. paper)
I. Title.   II. Series: Oxford American psychiatry library.
[DNLM: 1. Bipolar Disorder. WM 207]
RC516
616.89'5—dc23   2014001687

I would like to dedicate this book to my wife Stacy, my best friend since we were 16 and whose love and encouragement has supported me since we were kids!

Contents

Acknowledgments

The author thanks Dr. Melissa DelBello for reading most of this book and providing critical feedback and comments, particularly on the pediatric portions. He also thanks Dr. Cal Adler for his input. Finally, he is indebted to the outstanding help provided by his OUP team: David D'Addona, Meredith Keller and Divya Vasudevan.

O A P L
OXFORD AMERICAN PSYCHIATRY LIBRARY

Bipolar Disorder

Chapter 1

Introduction

In the past few years, it seems that almost monthly another celebrity—athlete, actor, or public figure—announces that they are struggling with bipolar disorder. The difficulties popular singer Britney Spears and *Superman* actress Margot Kidder experienced with bipolar illness received considerable attention because of the unfortunately public behavioral problems that they exhibited. Successful actress Catherine Zeta-Jones and Illinois Congressman Jesse Jackson Jr. both announced that they were receiving treatment for bipolar II disorder after being hospitalized; bipolar II disorder, prior to these announcements, was not typically known to the general public. Other celebrities ranging from comedian Ben Stiller to newscaster Jane Pauley to actress Carrie Fisher have discussed their struggles with bipolar disorder, helping to bring conversation to the shroud of mystery surrounding this mental illness. The courage of these popular and successful public figures to discuss their conditions helps to destigmatize bipolar disorder, even though oftentimes they were reluctant participants pushed to become public by an intrusive press. However, the apparent sudden increasing frequency of these announcements gives the misleading impression that bipolar disorder is somehow new or simply fashionable. Nothing could be further from the truth. Biblical and Greek writers described the key clinical components of bipolar disorder, namely mania and depression, thousands of years ago. For example, some scholars[1] now believe that Israel's first king, Saul, suffered from manic and depressive episodes, referred to as "evil spirits" and was initially treated with David's harp playing, which was, unfortunately, not effective for long:

> Now it came about on the next day that an evil spirit from God came mightily upon Saul and he raved in the midst of the house while David was playing the harp with his hand, as usual; and a spear was in Saul's hand. Saul hurled the spear for he thought "I will pin David to the wall." (1 Sam. 18:10–11)

This 3,000-year-old text, plus writings from other ancient sources that even more clearly identify individuals with mania and depression, tell us that bipolar disorder has accompanied humanity since the dawn of history, if not earlier. Moreover, Saul was not the only bipolar king in history as he is joined by a number of others (Table 1.1).[2,3]

Stigma and misconception historically limited public awareness about bipolar disorder until recently (and despite the increased press, both stigma and misconceptions still persist), but mental health practitioners and other healthcare providers experience 10–30% or more of their clinical practices comprised of bipolar patients. Bipolar disorders (type I and II) affect up to

Table 1.1 Selected Rulers with Bipolar Disorder[1-3]		
Leader	**Country**	**When Ruled**
King Saul	Israel	1049–1007 BC
King Charles IV	France	1322–1328 AD
King Charles XII	Sweden	1697–1718 AD
King George III	England	1760–1801 AD
Kaiser Wilhelm	Germany	1888–1918 AD

2–3% of the general population worldwide, making it more common than other well-recognized conditions like type 1 diabetes, rheumatoid arthritis, or HIV infection. Recent studies demonstrate that bipolar disorder is the sixth leading cause of disability worldwide and is associated with high rates of both morbidity and mortality; for example, death by suicide affects up to 15% of people with bipolar disorder.[2,4]

Although bipolar disorder represents a major public health problem, its causes remain incompletely understood. It is now clear that genetic factors play a significant role in the onset of bipolar disorder, as recent studies suggest a heritability risk of 85%.[5] Moreover, not only is bipolar disorder more common in family members of a bipolar proband, but so are other conditions, including major depressive and anxiety disorders. Unfortunately, the specific genes that cause bipolar disorder have not yet been identified. Moreover, it appears probable that genes confer a risk for bipolar disorder that then interacts with environmental effects, such as stress or substance abuse, to precipitate the illness. Bipolar disorder therefore appears to arise from dysregulation of prefrontal-limbic mood networks and may reflect underlying molecular abnormalities in mitochondrial energy management.[6] As the neurobiology of bipolar disorder is better defined, treatment advances will be able to move from the current reliance on strictly empirical and often serendipitous approaches to more targeted treatment development.

Although bipolar disorder is common in clinical settings, effectively managing bipolar disorder may be one of psychiatry's greatest challenges. The course of bipolar disorder is dynamic, with changes among mood states and complex combinations of symptoms that comprise these mood states. These changing, multifaceted symptom patterns complicate clinical assessment, so that it can be difficult to diagnose the illness. Even after the illness is diagnosed, its dynamic nature often leads clinicians, particularly inexperienced clinicians, on a wild ride of symptom chasing, rather than a deliberate program of illness management. The course of illness is further complicated by the common occurrence of a number of other medical and psychiatric conditions that themselves can be difficult to treat. These conditions include drug and alcohol abuse, anxiety disorders, attention deficit hyperactivity disorder (ADHD), migraine, and metabolic syndromes. Consequently, effective treatment of bipolar disorder is a challenge. Indeed, successful treatment is programmatic, incorporating sophisticated psychopharmacology, evidence-based therapies, lifestyle modifications, and general good health practices.

This Oxford American Psychiatry Library (OAPL) volume reviews practical and succinct descriptions of bipolar disorder and its management in order to provide a quick reference for the busy practitioner. This volume may also be useful for some patients and their families, as well as medical or psychology students who are trying to better understand this complex and sometimes mystifying condition. A major focus of this volume is to provide a programmatic approach to bipolar disorder management in order to eliminate the "symptom-chasing" approach that often leads to frequent unnecessary medication changes, excessive polypharmacy, and poor outcome. Ultimately, the goal of this volume is to improve the lives of people suffering from bipolar disorder.

[*Author's Note*: In this book I use the term "bipolar disorder" (singular form) to represent what is probably a group of conditions that perhaps more correctly would be called "bipolar disorders" (plural form). I made this choice because the singular form is more common in the vernacular; however, when distinctions among subtypes are important or relevant, I use the plural form.]

References

1. Ben-Noun L. What was the mental disease that afflicted King Saul? Clin Case Stud 2003; 2(4): 270–282.

2. Goodwin FK, Jamison KR. *Manic-Depressive Illness: Bipolar Disorders and Recurrent Depression*. 2nd ed. New York: Oxford University Press, 2007.

3. Jamison KR. *Touched with Fire*. New York: Free Press, 1993.

4. Narrow WE, Rae DS, Robins LN, Regier DA. Revised prevalence estimates of mental disorders in the United States: using a clinical significance criterion to reconcile two survey's estimates. Arch Gen Psychiatry 2002; 59:115–123.

5. Nurnberger JI Jr. Chapter 9: General genetics of bipolar disorder. In: SM Strakowski, ed., *The Bipolar Brain: Integrating Neuroimaging and Genetics*. New York: Oxford University Press, 2012.

6. Strakowski SM. Chapter 13: Integration and consolidation: A neurophysiological model of bipolar disorder. In: SM Strakowski, ed., *The Bipolar Brain: Integrating Neuroimaging and Genetics*. New York: Oxford University Press, 2012.

Chapter 2

Making a Diagnosis of Bipolar Disorder

2.1. Brief Historical Overview

As mentioned in Chapter 1, bipolar disorder is an ancient condition that has been described, in various forms, for centuries if not millennia. Nearly 3,000-year-old biblical writings depict depressive- and manic-like rages as expressions of "evil spirits."[1] The ancient Greeks recognized both depression (called "melancholia") and mania as medical conditions. Melancholia was believed to arise from an imbalance of humeral constituents, in particularly an excess of "black bile." Hippocrates (c. 400 BC) described the symptoms of melancholia to include prolonged despondency, loss of appetite, insomnia, and agitation—symptoms we still use today to diagnose major depression. The causes of mania were less clear to the ancients, perhaps "yellow bile," but the symptoms defining it seem very modern indeed: excessive energy "day and night," euphoria and irritability, grandiosity, and impetuous, impulsive, and aggressive behavior.[2]

Aretaeus of Cappadocia (c. AD 150) is credited with being the first to link mania with melancholia, hinting at the condition we now call bipolar disorder. From that time forward, writers explored connections between mania and melancholia, typically concluding that mania was simply a more severe form of melancholia or that one syndrome precipitated the other. The French psychiatrist Falret, in 1854, integrated the two mood states into a single cycling condition that he termed *la folie circulaire*; his contemporary Baillarger independently concluded virtually the same thing at the same time (*la folie a double forme*). This notion that melancholia and mania were different expressions or phases of an underlying cyclic illness remains the basis of how we think about bipolar disorder today. Emil Kraepelin advanced this French concept with his landmark descriptions and separation in 1899 of "dementia praecox," which roughly corresponds to what we now call schizophrenia, and "manic-depressive insanity." Kraepelin's distinction was largely based on outcome, in which manic-depressive insanity was associated with recovery, but dementia praecox was not. Kraepelin included what we would now call bipolar disorder plus recurrent major depression in the concept of manic-depressive insanity. This conceptualization was viewed as too broad by many psychiatrists, however, leading Leonhard in 1957 to coin the term "bipolar" to describe individuals who experienced mania and depression (i.e., two poles) as distinct from those with only recurrent major depression (i.e., one pole or "unipolar" depression).[2] Independent landmark studies by Angst

(1966),[3] Perris (1968),[4] and Winokur and Clayton (1967)[5] provided clinical and family history data supporting the bipolar-unipolar division of affective illnesses. As the use of lithium increased in the 1960s and 1970s, this classification of mood disorders was further supported, since lithium is relatively therapeutic for bipolar disorder, particularly mania, but not especially effective in the treatment of unipolar depression (or schizophrenia, for that matter). Although the symptoms and signs of bipolar disorder have been refined over the centuries, in fact, the core features of this condition were recognized throughout much of human history.

2.2. Mania and Hypomania

Bipolar disorder, then, is defined by the occurrence of mania or hypomania. Mania is defined by a euphoric, expansive, or irritable mood that is accompanied by a marked increase in energy. The symptoms must represent a change in the patient's typical behavior and must be relatively persistent for at least several days (e.g., at least one week in DSM-5).[6] Additionally, several other defining symptoms must be present to make a diagnosis of mania, the specific number of which varies according to the diagnostic criteria set but is typically three or more. These defining symptoms, listed in Box 2.1, serve as the basis for the two most widely used criteria sets, namely DSM-5 and ICD-10 (with ICD-11 "around the corner" and similar).[6,7] These same symptoms define hypomania. However, mania is diagnosed when these symptoms cause significant impairment in interpersonal, social, or work function; by definition, if someone requires hospitalization due to these symptoms, then mania is diagnosed. In contrast, hypomania is diagnosed when symptoms represent a significant change from the individual's typical behavior, but do not produce functional impairment. Other symptoms occurring during mania or hypomania, that are not necessarily required to make a diagnosis, but nonetheless are relatively frequent, are listed in Box 2.2.

The extreme mood state of mania or hypomania is not necessarily fixed every hour of every day of an episode; in fact, commonly affected individuals exhibit mood lability, demonstrating rapid shifts in mood from moment to moment that can range from euphoria to irritability and can include periods of depression. The excessive energy of mania may be purposefully directed

---

Box 2.1 Defining Symptoms of Mania

- Euphoric, expansive, or irritable mood
- Excessive energy
- Decreased need for sleep
- Racing thoughts/flight of ideas
- Rapid speech
- Grandiosity
- Impulsive pleasure seeking
- Distractibility

Box 2.2 Other Common Symptoms of Mania

- Mood lability
- Hypersexuality
- Brief periods of depressed mood
- Hallucinations
- Delusions
- Severe thought disorder
- Aggressive impulsivity
- Confusion
- Hyperreligiosity
- Extravagance
- Catatonia

---

toward projects, some of which might be quite grandiose (e.g., starting a rock band with no musical experience), or may simply be expressed as restlessness and agitation. This excessive psychomotor energy level is typically expressed in lack of need for sleep; manic individuals may go for several days with only a few hours or even no sleep. Manic individuals talk fast and think fast, although their conversation is often jumbled and loosely connected. Although in classic cases of mania, impulsivity is directed toward pleasurable, but risky, activities, aggressive and even violent impulsivity may also occur, particularly with irritable individuals. If left untreated, an episode of mania might persist for several months and can escalate into delirium, catatonia, and even death through dehydration and exhaustion. In the extreme, mania is a medical emergency requiring rapid intervention.

Mania is one of the most predictive syndromes in psychiatric. Following a single manic episode, the affected individual has an 80% risk of recurrent manic and depressive episodes consistent with a bipolar course of illness. Nonetheless, mania is still a nonspecific syndrome that can occur separately from bipolar disorder due to other medical causes that impact brain function. Some of these more common conditions are listed in Box 2.3. In these cases, the manic episode is commonly referred to as "secondary mania," that is, secondary to an underlying medical condition other than bipolar disorder.

> *Key Point*: Mania and hypomania are symptomatically similar, but differ by the greater functional impairment of mania. Mania predicts a bipolar life course in over 80% of individuals.

2.3. Bipolar Depression

Although mania or hypomania defines the diagnosis of bipolar disorder, in most cases depression also occurs during the course of illness. In fact, individuals with bipolar disorder typically spend more time in depression than mania, and depression is often the more disabling mood state.[8] The diagnosis

Box 2.3 Possible Medical Causes of Secondary Mania

Traumatic brain injury
Cerebrovascular disease
Brain tumors
Drug intoxication/withdrawal
Hyperthyroidism
CNS infections
Epilepsy
Huntington's disease
Dementia

Adapted from Sax and Strakowski[13]

of depression in bipolar individuals is no different from that in anyone else and relies on the same set of symptoms, listed in Box 2.4.

Despite its name, the most defining symptom of a major depressive episode is anhedonia, namely the loss of the ability to experience pleasure or a disinterest in pleasurable activities that a person would normally pursue. In some cultures, and often in men, depressed individuals will not complain about feeling down or sad, but will acknowledge anhedonia, often expressed as a loss of interest in sex. Of course, persistent despondency, sadness, and depressed mood are also commonly present and a defining symptom of a major depressive episode. Typically, depressed patients complain of low energy (in contrast to mania), which may be accompanied by moving and thinking more slowly (psychomotor retardation); agitation is also relatively common and can make distinguishing an agitated depression from a mixed state very difficult (for more on this topic, see section 2.4, "Bipolar Mixed States"). Concentration difficulties occur, although in depression these are more likely to be expressed as straightforward inattention, rather than the distractibility of mania. Neurovegetative signs include either increased or decreased sleep, appetite, and weight. Psychosis (hallucinations and delusions) and catatonia can occur during a severe depressive episode, as with mania.

The most concerning symptom of depression is suicidality; suicide is a horrendous permanent solution for a temporary (and almost always treatable)

Box 2.4 Defining Symptoms of Depression

- Depressed mood
- Anhedonia
- Feelings of worthlessness or excessive guilt
- Change in appetite and weight
- Psychomotor agitation or retardation
- Change in sleep pattern
- Fatigue
- Impaired concentration
- Suicidal thoughts or behavior

problem, the prevention of which is a major focus of treatment. Sadly, bipolar disorder has among the highest lifetime rates of suicide attempts (up to half of patients) and suicides (up to 15% of patients) of any medical condition. These attempts often occur during the depressed phase of illness, although they are particularly common in mixed states with the potential lethal combination of high energy concurrent with dysphoria and hopelessness.

Traditionally, two weeks of depressive symptoms are required to make a diagnosis of major depression.[6,7] As with mania, an episode of depression is not diagnosed unless it impairs psychosocial function. Depression is also a relatively common consequence of any medical condition that impacts brain function, including virtually every other psychiatric diagnosis. This so-called secondary depression is much more common than secondary mania.

Although the diagnostic criteria for bipolar and unipolar depression are the same, depressed bipolar individuals are more likely to express so-called atypical depression. Atypical depression includes hypersomnia instead of insomnia, weight gain instead of weight loss, psychomotor retardation rather than agitation, and mood lability within a depressive episode. Psychosis and catatonia may be more common in bipolar than unipolar depression as well. However, none of these depressive symptoms, alone or in combination, distinguish bipolar from unipolar depression; as noted, a diagnosis of bipolar disorder can only be made with the occurrence of mania or hypomania.

> *Key Point*: Bipolar and unipolar depression can only be differentiated by the occurrence of mania or hypomania in bipolar disorder.

2.4. Bipolar Mixed States

The "bipolar" nomenclature is somewhat misleading because it implies that affected individuals exist on two distinct poles, namely depression *or* mania and that these two poles never meet. In fact, in roughly one-half of episodes, depressive and manic symptoms occur concurrently. Despite mixed states being common, there has been ongoing controversy since Kraepelin about how to best define them. In DSM-IV,[9] a mixed state was only diagnosed when both the manic and depressive symptoms met full criteria for both episodes. In ICD-10,[7] they are identified by various combinations of manic and depressive symptoms (which will probably persist into ICD-11). In DSM-5,[6] mixed states have been replaced by a "mixed" modifier of either manic or depressive episodes, allowing the clinician more leeway in making this determination. These different approaches arise from the complexity of bipolar mood episodes, as many of the symptoms of mania and depression are similar and hence overlapping (e.g., poor concentration versus distractibility, decreased need for sleep versus insomnia). Moreover, depressive and dysphoric moods can occur even during "pure" mania as part of the mood lability of that condition. These mixed manic-depressive episodes are diagnostically challenging to recognize and may be less responsive to some treatment interventions. Specifically, mixed states appear to be less responsive to lithium than is mania; conversely, during antidepressant treatment mixed states may be more sensitive to manic switches than are "pure" depressive episodes. As noted earlier, mixed states appear to represent the affective phase with the highest risk for suicide, likely because of the combination of high energy and severely dysphoric mood and cognition.[10] Practically, then, when assessing mood states in bipolar patients, it is important to review the entire range of affective symptoms and signs, while carefully considering the potential impact of manic and depressive combinations on treatment planning.

2.5. Bipolar Disorder Subtypes

Given the symptom complexity of both mania and depression, it is not surprising that clinicians and psychiatric investigators have debated for decades, if not centuries, about whether there are subtypes of bipolar disorder that might have different treatment requirements and prognoses. Indeed, there is currently an active debate over whether these subtypes exist at all or whether there is a spectrum of manic or depressive symptoms in people that are not easily classified into categories. To date, there is no resolution of this debate, although the best evidence suggests two distinct bipolar conditions, namely bipolar I and bipolar II disorders, as well as a possibly related but less symptomatically severe condition called cyclothymia.[6,7]

Bipolar I disorder is the classic version of bipolar disorder, defined by the occurrence of mania. Although depression typically occurs during the course of bipolar I disorder, perhaps 10% of individuals only experience recurrent mania. However, the treatment, symptom expression, and familial patterns of this latter group do not differ substantially from those of individuals who experience both mania and depression, so they are classified together.

Bipolar II disorder is defined by the occurrence of at least one hypomanic episode as well as one or more depressive episodes. This subtype of bipolar disorder is relatively modern, not really being defined until the seminal work of Dunner and colleagues in the 1970s.[11] Bipolar II disorder differs from bipolar I disorder primarily by the level of functional impairment of the manic symptoms, although this difference should not be interpreted as bipolar II disorder being less impairing than bipolar I disorder. Indeed, in both bipolar subtypes, it is the more persistent depressive symptoms that impart the majority of the disability. Bipolar II disorder may also differ from bipolar I disorder by having more frequent mood changes with less time spent in euthymia. Individuals with bipolar II disorder may be more responsive to antidepressants than bipolar I disorder, although this difference is not well established. Bipolar II disorder may be genetically distinct from bipolar I disorder, supporting this categorical separation, although not all studies have been able to replicate this observation.

Cyclothymia is defined by the occurrence of significant mood changes that contain both manic and depressive features, but never meet criteria for full manic or depressive episodes. Some investigators and clinicians believe that cyclothymia is more accurately viewed as a temperament (i.e., a personality style) rather than an affective illness. In either case, it is typically chronic and can impart significant disability. In children who demonstrate cyclothymia, up to two-thirds appear to later develop bipolar disorder, whereas cyclothymia in adults is unlikely to progress. It appears, then, that cyclothymia is related differently to bipolar I and II disorders depending on when in an individual's life the condition occurs. Whether cyclothymia and bipolar I and II disorders are genetically related in adults remains unclear.

> *Key Point.* Bipolar I disorder is differentiated from bipolar II disorder by the presence of functional impairment associated with manic symptoms in the former.

2.6. Bipolar Spectrum

A number of psychiatric investigators and theorists have advocated for the notion of a bipolar spectrum. This spectrum might extend from minor depressive symptoms or dysthymia (chronic low-grade depression) through recurrent depressive episodes that gradually progress to the addition of increasing manic symptoms (e.g., cyclothymia) through full hypomania (bipolar II disorder) and mania (bipolar I disorder). Considerable focus has been on individuals with recurrent major depressive episodes, who are often treatment unresponsive and whose course of illness is accompanied by subclinical manic symptoms. In DSM-5 these patients are classified under Unspecified Bipolar Disorder, and in ICD-10 they are classified under Bipolar Affective Disorder Not Elsewhere Classified (NEC).[6,7] Unfortunately, few treatment and genetic data provide specific support for relationships among these conditions and the better recognized bipolar I and II disorders. At this time, then, the spectrum approach does not provide particularly useful guidance for treatment decisions, but may have heuristic value for refining diagnostic criteria in the future. That said, like cyclothymia, these nonspecific bipolar syndromes in children represent a risk for progression to bipolar I or II disorder, again suggesting a developmental aspect to symptom expression of bipolar illness across the life span.[12]

> *Key Point:* The concept of a bipolar spectrum defined by various combinations and severity of manic and depressive symptoms is insufficiently developed to guide clinical decision-making at this time.

2.7. Bipolar Disorder Course Progression and Patterns of Illness

As illustrated in Figure 2.1, psychiatric investigators have known for decades that the early course of bipolar disorder is progressive.[13] Specifically, following each major affective episode, the euthymic period until the next episode progressively shortens until the condition tends toward a relatively stable pattern of recurrences, typically annually if not treated or otherwise disrupted. An important caveat of Figure 2.1 is that this pattern of illness appears to be essentially the same in the pre- and postpharmacologic eras, raising questions

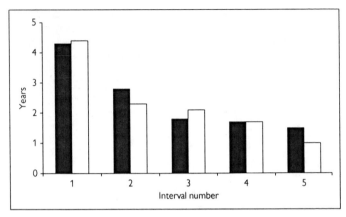

Figure 2.1 Chart illustrating decreasing length of intervals between successive affective episodes. (Source: Dark bar = data from Kraepelin 1921 cited in Strakowski 2012; light bar = data from Roy-Byrne et al. 1985 cited in Strakowski 2012. Adapted from Strakowski 2012).[13]

about how effectively our treatments ultimately impact this progression. As will be discussed in Chapter 5, it is likely that this progressive shortening of euthymic intervals in bipolar disorder reflects an underlying progressive neuropathology that leads from a single manic episode to a recurring affective illness.

Also as illustrated in Figure 2.1, because the length of euthymic intervals progressively shortens, the well interval after a first manic episode can be relatively long, on average up to 3-4 years. This relatively long interval often misleads affected individuals and their care providers into thinking that their manic episode was a one-time event, so that most of these individuals drop out of treatment based on a false assumption that they will never again experience mania. Unfortunately, an episode of mania predicts a long-term bipolar course of illness, that is, recurrent manic and depressive episodes, more than 80% of the time, so that the vast majority of these individuals relapse. Understanding the predictive power of mania coupled with the progressive nature of bipolar disorder becomes important to guide young individuals and their families into realistic expectations about this condition.

Although mania and hypomania define bipolar I and II disorders respectively, and are relatively more dramatic than depression, nonetheless depressive symptoms dominate the course of bipolar illness. In a long-term, large study of bipolar patients supported by the National Institute of Mental Health (NIMH), investigators found that over a period of 13 years, individuals with bipolar disorder spent 32% of the time with depressive symptoms, compared with 9% of the time with manic symptoms and 6% of the time with mixed symptoms.[8] Depression is also associated with most of the functional impairment of bipolar disorder. Indeed, mania can be quite disruptive to people's lives, but it is relatively short-lived, a few weeks or months at most even without treatment. In contrast, depression can persist for months or even years and truly become crippling. Moreover, bipolar depression can be quite a challenge to treat, as it is relatively less responsive to standard antidepressant pharmacotherapy than unipolar major depression; we will discuss the management of bipolar depression in Chapter 7.

As noted, the typical course of bipolar disorder, if unmanaged, will often settle into an annual cycle of mania followed or preceded by depression. However, some individuals develop rapid cycling, typically defined as four or more distinct affective episodes within a single year. Rapid cycling can be very difficult to treat, although it appears to generally be time limited and is probably initiated by a specific psychosocial or biological trigger. Common precipitants for rapid cycling include drug or alcohol abuse, major life stressors, thyroid disease or other new medical illness, and exposure to new medications. Women appear to be more likely to develop rapid cycling, which is also more common in bipolar II than bipolar I disorder (see Chapter 8).

Some individuals may also develop chronic affective symptoms that switch between mania and depression, but never achieve euthymic periods. In children and adolescents with bipolar disorder, mood symptoms are commonly expressed as chronic affective instability with few distinct manic or depressive episodes. In these young people, making a diagnosis can be challenging and is typically suggested by the presence of this affective instability coupled with a family history of bipolar disorder. However, in these young individuals, a specific diagnosis of bipolar I or II disorder may not be possible for many years, until they are old enough to express a clear manic or hypomanic episode (see Chapter 8).

2.8. Differential Diagnosis of Bipolar Disorder

A number of conditions share symptoms with bipolar disorder, so must be ruled out when making the diagnosis. Common conditions that may be confused with bipolar disorder include:

Recurrent major depression: As noted, individuals suffering from bipolar disorder spend much of their course of illness with depressive symptoms and syndromes, such that the manic or hypomanic episodes are relatively rare. Distinguishing bipolar individuals from those who only experience recurrent major depression can be difficult and is completely dependent upon identifying manic or hypomanic episodes.

Dysthymia: Dysthymia is a condition characterized by chronic depressive symptoms that do not achieve the level of a major depressive syndrome (episode). It is not uncommon for individuals with bipolar disorder to exhibit these types of subsyndromal symptoms of depression between major affective episodes. Again, a diagnosis of bipolar disorder cannot be made until the occurrence of mania or hypomania. Dysthymia and cyclothymia can also be difficult to distinguish, as both experience subsyndromal depression; however, individuals with cyclothymia also exhibit subsyndromal symptoms of mania.

Schizophrenia: Schizophrenia is a complex condition characterized by chronic psychotic symptoms, personality deterioration, and typically profound functional impairment. Most people with schizophrenia also experience episodes of depression. Psychosis commonly occurs during manic episodes and can also occur with depression during the course of bipolar disorder, which contributes to the confusion between these conditions. However, bipolar disorder with psychotic features can be differentiated from schizophrenia by identifying affective symptoms that are more prominent and common than the co-occurring psychosis. Additionally, psychosis in bipolar disorder is primarily restricted to affective episodes, whereas in schizophrenia, psychosis is persistent independent of affective symptoms.

Schizoaffective disorder, bipolar type: Individuals suffering from schizoaffective disorder, bipolar type, exhibit both mania and depression that is relatively prominent throughout the course of illness, yet also experience periods of psychosis independent of affective symptoms. This diagnostic category is somewhat controversial, and many psychiatric investigators (including the author) consider schizoaffective disorder, bipolar-type to simply represent an extreme form of bipolar I disorder. Indeed, treatment of this condition is virtually the same as for bipolar I disorder.

Borderline personality disorder: Individuals suffering from borderline personality disorder exhibit chronic mood instability, tempestuous interpersonal relationships, self-destructive and often chronic suicidal behavior, and impulsivity. The onset is typically gradual, emerging from a lifelong disturbance in interpersonal relationships. Bipolar disorder is distinguished from borderline personality disorder by the occurrence of distinct, affective episodes (particularly mania), periods of euthymia, and often a relatively distinct age at onset. However, these two conditions can be very difficult to differentiate at times, particularly in adolescents. Moreover, these conditions are not mutually exclusive, so may co-occur. Whereas bipolar disorder is equally common between sexes, borderline personality disorder is more common in women. It also appears to be more commonly associated with a history of childhood physical and sexual abuse than bipolar disorder.

Attention Deficit Hyperactivity Disorder (ADHD): ADHD is characterized by distractibility, impulsive behavior, and excessive energy similar to the symptoms of mania or hypomania. However, in ADHD these symptoms tend to be relatively persistent and chronic, whereas in bipolar disorder, they present within episodes of mania or hypomania. Bipolar disorder is further distinguished from ADHD by the occurrence of affective episodes. By definition, ADHD begins prior to age 7 years, whereas the onset of bipolar disorder is typically in the teens. Diagnoses of ADHD and bipolar disorder are not mutually exclusive and commonly co-occur in younger patients. Moreover, in youth with a family history of bipolar disorder, the onset of ADHD may predict the emergence of bipolar illness at a later age.

Drug/alcohol use disorders: Chronic drug or alcohol use is commonly associated with mood instability and behavioral dyscontrol that might resemble the symptoms of bipolar disorder. Many drugs of abuse (e.g., alcohol) specifically produce depressive symptoms. Stimulants can produce symptoms that look like mania. Further complicating this differential is that drug and alcohol abuse occurs in more than half of individuals with bipolar disorder at some point in their lives. Bipolar disorder can be differentiated from affective illness secondary to substance abuse by occurrence of affective symptoms during periods of sobriety, onset of affective symptoms prior to the onset of substance abuse, or rapid resolution of affective symptoms following acute detoxification.

Other neurological and medical illnesses: Although depression is a common, nonspecific response to nearly any condition that impacts brain function, mania is a relatively rare event outside of bipolar disorder. Nonetheless, a number of medical conditions that impact brain function have been associated with mania and are listed in Box 2.5.[14] A first onset of mania after age 50 always warrants a careful medical evaluation to rule out conditions such as those listed in Box 2.5. Some of these conditions are more common in bipolar than in healthy individuals as well, which will be discussed in more detail in Chapter 3.

> *Key Point*: A number of medical and psychiatric conditions resemble bipolar disorder, but can typically be distinguished by a lack of clear manic or hypomanic episodes and an absence of a family history of bipolar disorder.

Box 2.5 Examples of Medical Causes of Mania

- Head trauma
- Neurological abnormalities
    - Stroke or brain hemorrhage
    - Multiple sclerosis
    - Brain cancer or tumors
    - Cerebral sarcoidosis
    - Tuberous sclerosis
    - Temporal lobe epilepsy
    - Huntington's disease
- Metabolic diseases
    - Hyperthyroidism
    - Cushing's disease
    - Wilson's disease
- CNS infection
    - Neurosyphilis
    - HIV/AIDS
- Other illnesses
    - CNS lupus
    - Klinefelter's syndrome

Adapted from Sax & Strakowski 1999[14]

References

1. Ben-Noun L. What was the mental disease that afflicted King Saul? Clin Case Stud 2003; 2(4): 270–282.

2. Angst J, Marneros A. Bipolarity from ancient to modern times: conception, birth and rebirth. J Aff Disord 2001; 67:3–19.

3. Angst J. *Zur Atiologie und Nosologie endogener depressiver Psychnose.* Berlin: Springer-Verlag, 1966.

4. Perris C. The course of depressive psychoses. Acta Psychiatr Scand 1968; 44(3):238–248.

5. Winokur G, Clayton P. Family history studies: I. Two types of affective disorders separated according to genetic and clinical factors. In: Worris J, ed., *Recent Advances in Biological Psychiatry* (Vol 10), pp. 35–50. New York: Plenum Press, 1976.

6. American Psychiatry Association. Diagnostic and Statistical Manual of Mental Health Disorders (5th edition). Washington, DC: American Psychiatric Press, 2012.

7. World Health Organization. ICD-10 Classifications of Mental and Behavioural Disorder: Clinical Descriptions and Diagnostic Guidelines. Geneva: World Health Organization, 1992.

8. Judd LL, Akiskal HS, Schettler PJ, Endicott J, Maser J, Solomon DA, Leon AC, Rice JA, Keller MB. The long-term natural history of the weekly symptomatic status of bipolar I disorder. Arch Gen Psychiatry 2002; 59:530–537.

9. American Psychiatric Association. Diagnostic and Statistical Manual of Mental Health Disorders (4th ed.). Washington DC: American Psychiatric Press, 1994.

10. Strakowski SM, McElroy SL, Keck PE Jr., West SA. Suicidality among patients with mixed and manic bipolar disorder. Am J Psychiatry 1996; 153:674–676.

11. Dunner DL, Gershon ES, Goodwin FK. Heritable factors in the severity of affective illness. Biol Psychiatry 1976; 11:31–42.

12. Strakowski SM, Fleck DE, Maj M. Broadening the diagnosis of bipolar disorder: benefits vs. risks. World Psychiatry 2011; 10:181–186.

13. Strakowski SM. Chapter 13: Integration and consolidation: a neurophysiological model of bipolar disorder. In: SM Strakowski, ed., *The Bipolar Brain: Integrating Neuroimaging and Genetics.* New York: Oxford University Press, 2012.

14. Sax KW, Strakowski SM. Chapter 8: The Co-occurrence of bipolar disorder with medical illness. In: Tohen M, ed. *Comorbidity in Affective Disorders.* New York: Marcel Dekker, 1999.

Chapter 3

Epidemiology of Bipolar Disorder

3.1. Population Prevalence and Incidence

Bipolar disorder is relatively common; the specific prevalence of bipolar disorder depends in part on the definition applied, whether bipolar I and II disorders are differentiated, and whether bipolar "spectrum" conditions are included. Nonetheless, rates of bipolar I disorder have been identified through several recent, large-scale epidemiologic studies that, despite some variability, converge around a lifetime prevalence rate of 1–1.5% (Table 3.1).[1-4] Rates for bipolar II disorder are more variable, although the National Comorbidity Survey-Revised (NCS-R) found it to be similar to bipolar I disorder, namely 1.1%.[3] Other studies find bipolar II disorder to be slightly less common than bipolar I disorder. These rates appear to be relatively consistent across countries and cultures with cross-national studies suggesting a range from lows in Iceland and Asia of around 0.2% to highs in the Netherlands of around 2.0%.[4-6] Consistent with this observation, in a review of a number of European studies, rates of bipolar I disorder were typically in the range of 1.3–1.8% with rates of bipolar II disorder similar, although perhaps slightly lower.[5] Whether these cross-national differences reflect "true" differences in rates or instead differences in methods and case ascertainment is not clear, but it is reasonable to conclude that bipolar disorders are similarly prevalent worldwide.

As described in Chapter 2, in recent years there has been increasing interest in the concept of a bipolar spectrum, that is, a spectrum of illness that extends from minor depressive symptoms through recurrent depressive episodes that gradually progress with the addition of increasing symptoms to mania (bipolar I disorder). Several attempts have been made to identify the prevalence of people who exhibit depression and manic symptoms who never meet criteria for bipolar I or II disorders. Because there is no agreed upon definition for these subthreshold "bipolar" cases, studies of the rates of people with these conditions are somewhat controversial and variable. Nonetheless, the NCS-R reported a rate of bipolar disorder spectrum of 4.5%, with over half of those representing subthreshold cases.[3] In the World Mental Health survey initiative, the rate of bipolar spectrum was 4.8%, with nearly three-fourths of the subjects expressing subthreshold or spectrum diagnoses, rather than bipolar I or II disorders.[6] Even higher rates were suggested in several European studies, as bipolar spectrum conditions were noted to occur in approximately 6% of the population.[5] The validity of the bipolar spectrum remains to be established, but these studies suggest that

Table 3.1 Rates of Bipolar I Disorder in Epidemiological Studies	
Study	**Prevalence (%)**
ECA, 1980	0.9
NCS, 1990	1.7
NCS-R, 2005	1.0
CNCG, 1996	0.5-1.5

ECA = Epidemiologic Catchment Area study;[1] NCS = National Comorbidity Survey;[2] NCS-R = National Comorbidity Survey-Revised;[3] CNCG = Cross-National Collaborative Group.[4]

bipolar-like conditions may be more common than currently thought using existing criteria sets.

> *Key Point*: Bipolar disorder is common, with types I and II affecting 1–3% of the population worldwide; less well defined spectrum conditions may increase that rate to 6%.

3.2. Subgroups and Other Factors

3.2.1. Gender

Unlike depressive disorders in which women are two to three times more likely to be diagnosed than men, bipolar disorder appears to be similarly distributed between the sexes. For example, in the National Comorbidity Survey, lifetime rates of bipolar I disorder in men and women were 1.6% and 1.7% respectively; in the NCS-R, these rates were 0.8% and 1.1%.[2,3] Similar types of sex distributions were noted in cross-national studies, suggesting that this equal risk extends across nations and cultures.[4–6]

The sex distribution of bipolar II disorder is less clear, but again lifetime rates appear to be similar between men and women. For example, in the NCS-R, men and women demonstrated similar lifetime rates of 0.9% and 1.3% respectively.[3] Although data are sparse, the less well defined bipolar spectrum also appears to demonstrate similar rates across the sexes.

> *Key Point*: Men and women are equally likely to develop bipolar disorder.

3.2.2. Age Effects

Bipolar disorder starts during youth and then persists across the life span. Studies of bipolar I disorder have largely converged toward a median age at onset in the range of 18–22 years across a variety of survey methods, countries, and ethnic/racial groups.[1] Although less well studied, bipolar II disorder also appears to commonly begin in adolescence. Consequently, we now know that most individuals who develop bipolar disorder begin experiencing symptoms in adolescence or even younger. Unfortunately, individuals with bipolar disorder are not correctly diagnosed on average for 7–10 years. In particular, hypomanic episodes are often not recognized in bipolar II disorder, leading to frequent misdiagnoses of recurrent major depression and then years of multiple ineffective antidepressant trials. Mania with psychosis (i.e., bipolar I disorder) is frequently misdiagnosed as schizophrenia; this risk is particularly high for individuals of African descent (discussed in the next section).[7,8] Consequently, although onset typically occurs in adolescence, recognition of bipolar illness often does not occur until the 20s, leading to a false impression by many clinicians of a later age at onset of these conditions than is actually correct.

Diagnosing bipolar disorder in the early teens or in preadolescents is controversial since, as mentioned in Chapter 2, it is relatively uncommon for these individuals to present with manic or hypomanic episodes that meet standard adult criteria (e.g., DSM-5, ICD-10). Studies of children at risk for bipolar disorder suggest that, prior to mid-to-late adolescence, the condition may be more chronic and continuous, rather than episodic, so that they often receive spectrum diagnoses (e.g., Unspecified Bipolar Disorder in DSM-5). Uncertainty in the manner in which bipolar disorder presents in youth challenges attempts to identify the specific prevalence rates. In the NCS study, the rate of bipolar I disorder in 15- to 17-year-old individuals was 1.4%, similar to that in adults.[2] This finding is inconsistent with a median onset of 18 years, since, based on that median, the prevalence in the younger age range should be less than half of that in adults. In the ECA study, when respondents were divided into 10-year cohorts, there was a progressive increase in rates of bipolar disorder across generations beginning with individuals born in the 1930s.[1] These findings raise the question of whether bipolar disorder is becoming more prevalent over time; that is, increasing rates with each generation, the so-called birth cohort effect. However, given that bipolar disorder has been described and recognized as common for millennia, it seems unlikely that there has been a substantial increase with each generation, since that would have produced a much higher rate than we currently observe. Moreover, given the controversy around diagnosis in younger people, it seems more likely that these age effects during the past century reflect changes in how bipolar disorder is identified and reflects an increased awareness of the condition in general. Indeed, other studies have found lifetime rates of bipolar disorder in adolescents to be much less than adult rates, as would be predicted in the absence of birth cohort effects. Clearly, much remains to be learned about how bipolar disorder presents in young patients, and how it evolves and progresses prior to the first manic episode.

> *Key Point*: Bipolar disorder typically begins in mid-adolescence to early adulthood. Once a manic or hypomanic episode has occurred, most individuals will experience a life-long course of bipolar illness, that is, recurring manic and depressive episodes.

3.3.3. Race/Ethnicity

As noted previously, rates of bipolar disorder are approximately the same across a wide range of countries and cultures. Within the United States, a number of studies have examined the impact of ethnic or racial designation on rates of bipolar disorder, with a primary focus on contrasts between white and African American subjects. Typically, once other demographic differences are controlled, epidemiological studies have not found racial differences in rates of bipolar disorder between these two groups. One exception to that observation was that the NCS reported lower rates of affective disorders in general and mania specifically in African American compared to white individuals; however, this racial difference in bipolar disorder rates was not observed in the NCS-R.[2,3]

In contrast to epidemiologic studies, for decades investigators observed that darker-skinned individuals of African descent in the United States and western Europe appeared to receive excessive clinical diagnoses of schizophrenia with lower rates of bipolar and other affective disorders. In particular, African Americans with mood disorders are two to nine times more likely to be diagnosed with schizophrenia than otherwise similar white individuals in clinical settings. Similar diagnostic differences are observed in Afro-Caribbeans in the UK. Several studies suggest that in these individuals, clinicians overemphasize psychotic symptoms and minimize affective symptoms, leading to misidentification of mood disorders as schizophrenia. More careful application of diagnostic criteria, for example, through the use of structured interviews, seems to improve this problem, although does not correct it entirely. Some of the difficulty may reflect cultural differences in "idioms of distress," that is, how individuals from different ethnic backgrounds describe their behavioral symptoms. Regardless, this literature reminds clinicians to be sensitive to differences in symptom expression among multicultural groups when assigning a diagnosis.[7,8]

> Key Point: African Americans with bipolar disorder are at high risk for being clinically misdiagnosed with schizophrenia.

3.3. Burden of Disease

3.3.1. Morbidity and Disability

Bipolar disorder is typically a lifelong illness for which there is no known cure. Although a number of treatments decrease the frequency and duration of episodes, there is no known intervention that prevents all new episodes. Consequently, individuals with bipolar disorder struggle with affective and cognitive symptoms throughout their lives.

A number of longer-term outcome studies examined the course of illness in individuals with bipolar disorder; these studies ranged from 1 to 40 years in duration. Once a first manic episode occurs, more than 90% of individuals will progress to a life-long bipolar illness; namely, recurrent manic, hypomanic, and depressive episodes. In the 40-year Zurich outcome study, Angst and Preiseg[9] observed that 16% of individuals essentially recover with relatively minimal symptoms, whereas another 16% are chronically ill; therefore, two-thirds of individuals with bipolar disorder struggle with recurrent symptoms, but manage to achieve some periods of euthymia. As described in Chapter 2, the bulk of the time with symptoms is spent in depression. Recovery from symptoms appears to be most likely early in the course of illness, and subsyndromal symptoms are typical after several episodes.

Symptom recovery is only a part of the picture, as, even as symptoms resolve following an acute affective episode, functional impairment persists for many months. The University of Cincinnati outcome studies[10] found that during the first year following an acute manic episode, more than 75% of individuals struggled with psychosocial function, unable to return to previous levels of employment, social function, or relationships; these impairments occurred even after the first manic episode, and these findings were similar to those from several other studies. Moreover, as discussed in Chapter 4, individuals with bipolar disorder suffer from higher rates of a wide range of other medical illnesses, and their lives are often complicated by co-occurring drug and alcohol use disorders that further worsen outcome. Indeed, bipolar disorder is recognized as one of the leading causes of medical disability worldwide, often among the top 10 most disabling conditions.

> *Key Point*: Bipolar disorder is a recurrent condition that is among the leading medical causes of disability worldwide. Functional impairment from bipolar disorder often persists for months after symptoms have resolved.

3.3.2. Mortality and Suicide

Individuals with bipolar disorder have higher rates of premature death than the general population at virtually every age. Although suicide is a major component of this increased risk, individuals with bipolar disorder also exhibit higher rates of a variety of medical illnesses contributing to this increased risk (see Chapter 4). In particular, individuals with bipolar disorder have a risk of premature mortality from cardiovascular disease that is two to three times higher than that of the general population. This risk likely reflects the very high rates of smoking (up to 80% in some studies), obesity, type II diabetes, and unhealthy lifestyles (e.g., drug and alcohol use disorders) that occur in bipolar disorder, although there may also be cardiovascular risks inherent to bipolar illness. Consequently, individuals with bipolar disorder die from medical illnesses at younger ages than their unaffected counterparts in the general population.[12]

Suicide is a common consequence of bipolar disorder. Up to 15% of individuals with bipolar disorder commit suicide, with the risk highest in the first 5–10 years of illness. Up to half of bipolar individuals will make a suicide attempt, with women more likely to do so than men, although completion rates are similar between the sexes (in contrast to the general population, in which men are more likely to complete suicide than women). Mixed mood states, drug and alcohol abuse, inadequate treatment, and co-occurring anxiety disorders increase the risk of suicide. Suicide may be more likely in the spring, perhaps reflecting seasonal variation in mood state, with switches from depression to mania or mixed states occurring at that time of year in many individuals. The strongest predictor of suicide is a history of previous suicide attempts.

Preventing suicide remains difficult. Although risk factors may be useful to predict the behavior of groups, they are often difficult to apply to a specific individual at a specific time. Treatment of suicidal individuals with bipolar disorder is discussed in more detail in Chapter 8.

> *Key Point*: Individuals with bipolar disorder have higher mortality rates than their peers from the general population, and suicide is a major contributor to this increased risk.

References

1. Weissman MM, Bruce ML, Leaf PJ, Florio LP, Holzer C. Affective disorders. In: Robins LN, Regier DA, eds. *Psychiatric Disorders in America: The Epidemiologic Catchment Area Study*, pp. 53–80. New York: Free Press, 1991.

2. Kessler RC, McGonagle KA, Zhao S, Nelson CB, Hughes M, Eshleman S, Wittchen HU, Kendler KS. Lifetime and 12-month prevalence of DSM-III-R psychiatric disorders in the United States. Results from the National Comorbidity Survey. Arch Gen Psychiatry 1994; 51:8–19.

3. Merikangas KR, Akiskal HS, Angst J, Greenberg PE, Hirschfeld RM, Petukhova M, Kessler RC. Lifetime and 12-month prevalence of bipolar spectrum disorder in the National Comorbidity Survey replication. Arch Gen Psychiatry. 2007; 64(5): 543–552.

4. Weissman MM, Bland RC, Canino GJ, Faravelli C, Greenwald S, Hwu H-G, Joyce PR, Karam EG, Lee C-K, Lellouch J, Lepine J-P, Newman SC, Rubio-Stipec M, Wells E, Wickramaratne PJ, Wittchen H-U, Yeh E-K. Cross-national epidemiology of major depression and bipolar disorder. JAMA 1996; 276:293–299.

5. Pini S, de Queiroz V, Pagnin D, Pezawas L, Angst J, Cassano GV, Wittchen H-U. Prevalence and burden of bipolar disorder in European countries. Euro Neuropsychopharm 2005; 15:425–434.

6. Merikangas KR, Jin R, He JP, Kessler RC, Lee S, Sampson NA, Viana MC, Andrade LH, Hu C, Karam EG, Ladea M, Medina-Mora ME, Ono Y, Posada-Villa J, Sagar R, Wells JE, Zarkov Z. Prevalence and correlates of bipolar spectrum disorder in the world mental health survey initiative. Arch Gen Psychiatry 2011;68:241–251.

7. Strakowski SM, Keck PE Jr., Arnold LM, Collins J, Wilson R, Fleck DE, Corey KB, Amicone J, Adebimpe VR. Ethnicity and diagnosis in patients with affective psychoses. J Clin Psychiatry 2003; 64:747–754.

8. Gara MA, Vega WA, Arndt S, Escamilla M, Fleck DE, Lawson WB, Lesser I, Neighbors HW, Wilson DR, Arnold LM, Strakowski SM. Influence of patient race and ethnicity on clinical assessment in patients with affective disorders. Arch Gen Psychiatry 2012; 69:593–600.

9. Angst J, Preisig M. Course of a clinical cohort of unipolar, bipolar and schizoaffective patients: results of a prospective study from 1959 to 1985. Schweiz Arch Neurol Psychiatr 1995;146:5–23.

10. Keck PE Jr., McElroy SL, Strakowski SM, West SA, Sax KW, Hawkins JM, Bourne ML, Haggard P. 12- month outcome of patients with bipolar disorder following hospitalization for a manic or mixed episode. Am J Psychiatry 1998; 155:646–652.

11. Goodwin FK, Jamison KR. Chapter 25: Clinical management of suicide risk. In: Goodwin FK, Jamison KR, eds., *Manic-Depressive Illness: Bipolar Disorders and Recurrent Depression*. New York: Oxford University Press, 2007.

Chapter 4

Illness Comorbidity and Co-occurrence in Bipolar Disorders

4.1. What Is Comorbidity?

In medical parlance, "comorbidity" refers to the occurrence of two or more medical conditions concurrently. Strictly defined, comorbidity requires that these conditions be independent. For example, if someone with coronary artery disease develops streptococcal pharyngitis, then these two illnesses are etiologically unrelated, so are comorbid. It is expected that a person with any one illness will develop second unrelated illnesses at essentially the base population rate. In contrast, if an individual with coronary artery disease experiences a stroke, then these conditions share an underlying vascular etiology. In this case, the second condition occurs at a rate higher than population base rates because it shares risk factors with the primary illness. Although this latter situation is often called comorbidity, technically that is a misuse of the term. Consequently, the term "co-occurrence" is often more accurate.

Because the specific etiology of bipolar disorder is unknown, defining comorbidity is relatively difficult, although secondary illnesses occurring at population base rates and that are unrelated to the central nervous system (e.g., again, streptococcal pharyngitis) likely meet the strict definition. Individuals with bipolar disorder are not protected from illnesses that affect the general population. However, bipolar individuals exhibit a number of conditions at elevated rates that suggest common etiologies or risk factors.

> *Key Point*: The course of bipolar disorder is commonly complicated by co-occurring medical and psychiatric conditions.

4.2. Co-occurring Psychiatric Illnesses

A number of psychiatric conditions occur in bipolar disorder at rates much higher than in the general population and are particularly relevant as they can confound illness management and, typically, worsen illness course. These conditions are listed in Table 4.1.

Table 4.1 Psychiatric Conditions Co-occurring with Bipolar Disorder

Condition	Lifetime Prevalence Bipolar Disorder	Lifetime Prevalence General Population
Alcohol use disorders	38–48%[1]	14–18%
Nicotine use disorders	46–80%	21%
Drug use disorders	21–41%[1]	6–8%
Anxiety disorders	42–77%	15–25%
Personality disorders	38–48%	9–13%
ADHD	28–90%[2]	5–10%

[1] Higher in bipolar I than bipolar II disorder
[2] Higher in younger individuals with bipolar disorder

4.2.1. Alcohol Use Disorders

Individuals with bipolar disorder exhibit high rates of alcohol abuse, affecting up to half of people at some point in their life. This rate is three to four times higher than in the general population. We proposed four hypotheses for this common co-occurrence.[1–3]

Hypothesis 1. The symptoms of bipolar disorder (e.g., impulsivity of mania) lead to increased alcohol use. However, studies typically do not support a close temporal association between alcohol use and affective symptoms, suggesting this hypothesis is probably incorrect in general, although it may be true for some individuals.

Hypothesis 2. Historically, clinicians assumed that alcohol abuse was an attempt by bipolar individuals to self-medicate symptoms, for example, insomnia or anxiety. As noted, course of illness data for both conditions do not demonstrate strong temporal links, so do not support this assumption in general, although, again, this association may occur in some individuals.

Hypothesis 3. Some investigators proposed that alcohol abuse causes bipolar disorder. Age at onset findings suggest that alcohol abuse commonly precedes the onset of mania in many individuals. Moreover, some studies suggest that premorbid alcoholism may be present in individuals whose bipolar illness begins later, and who have less family history of bipolar disorder. Consequently, alcoholism may be necessary to initiate bipolar illness in these individuals with an otherwise lower familial risk. How alcohol abuse might precipitate bipolar illness is not known.

Hypothesis 4. Rather than alcohol directly causing bipolar disorder, the final hypothesis suggests that alcohol use and bipolar disorders share risk factors. For example, a genetic tendency toward impulsive decision-making might increase the likelihood of both conditions. Family studies are inconclusive that this shared risk factor is genetic, so there may be environmental factors contributing to the risk as well or perhaps an interaction of environmental factors and genetics. Stress, for example, has been associated with precipitating affective episodes in bipolar disorder and relapses in alcohol abuse, so it could be such a factor. Unfortunately data to identify these risk factors are lacking.

At this point, then, none of these hypotheses singularly explains the excessive co-occurrence of bipolar and alcohol use disorders. It appears most likely that this co-occurrence accumulates from all of these proposed associations and perhaps others not yet identified. Regardless of the specific reasons for the common co-occurrence of bipolar and alcohol use disorders, alcohol abuse clearly worsens the course of bipolar illness. Alcohol abuse is associated with impaired treatment response, increased time in depression, increased risk of suicide, and worse functional outcome. Consequently, clinicians must be diligent for evidence of alcohol abuse in individuals with bipolar disorder, particularly when treatment response or course suddenly worsens. Once identified, both alcohol use and bipolar disorders must be managed aggressively; recent studies suggest that concurrent management using best practices for both conditions likely produces the best outcomes (Chapter 8).

4.2.2. Nicotine Use Disorders

The negative health consequences of cigarette smoking are well known, and, unfortunately, smoking is common in bipolar disorder, affecting up to 80% of individuals.[4] Despite being common, the impact of smoking on the course of bipolar disorder is not well studied, although in the general population cigarette use is associated with increased anxiety and suicide in addition to cancer, stroke, and heart disease and there is no reason to think *a priori* that these effects would be lessened by the presence of bipolar disorder. Moreover, not only is cigarette use more common in bipolar disorder, bipolar individuals are less successful at quitting. The reasons for this common co-occurrence are not known, although it likely occurs from accumulation of the hypothesized associations discussed for alcohol abuse. Given the negative health effects of cigarette use, it is imperative to aggressively address this co-occurrence in the management of bipolar disorder.

4.2.3. Other Drug Use Disorders

In addition to elevated abuse of "legal" drugs (nicotine and alcohol), there is also an excess of illicit and prescription drug use in bipolar disorder.[1–3] As noted in Table 4.1, the lifetime prevalence of drug abuse in bipolar disorder is three to six times greater than in the general population. The types of drugs most commonly abused reflect general population patterns of drug use with cannabis being most common; there is no convincing evidence that bipolar individuals are differentially selective of drugs of abuse. Again, the reasons for increased rates of drug abuse are unknown, but are likely similar to those for alcohol abuse. Regardless of the reasons, drug abuse significantly worsens the course of bipolar disorder, with increased affective episodes, poor psychosocial recovery and higher rates of suicide. Consequently, clinicians must closely monitor for drug abuse, particularly with sudden course changes. Alcohol and drug abuse, including cigarette smoking, often occur together requiring attention to all of them concurrently.

> *Key Point*: Co-occurring substance use disorders, including smoking, are very common and worsen the course of bipolar illness. These conditions should be managed concurrently with best practices for each to optimize illness outcome.

4.2.4. Anxiety Disorders

Anxiety occurs throughout the course of illness in most bipolar individuals, across all mood states, and even during periods of relative euthymia. Reflecting this high rate of anxiety *symptoms*, anxiety *disorders* are three to four times more common in bipolar disorder than in the general population (Table 4.2).[3,5] Increased rates across the spectrum of anxiety disorders in bipolar disorder have been reported. However, most consistently, studies report excessive co-occurrence of obsessive-compulsive disorder (OCD), panic disorder, and post-traumatic stress disorder (PTSD). The presence of anxiety disorders worsens the course of bipolar illness. Aggressive management of the primary bipolar condition will often alleviate anxiety symptoms, but anxiety disorders typically require additional treatment. Moreover, treating these conditions can be complicated, since anxiety disorders are typically managed with antidepressant medications that are not always tolerated by bipolar individuals. Consequently, alternative therapies (e.g., cognitive behavioral therapy) may need to be relied on more extensively (see Chapter 8). Of particular note, following the 9/11 attacks on New York, bipolar individuals were among the most likely to develop PTSD.[6] Consequently, individuals with bipolar disorder appear to be particularly susceptible to PTSD, so should be carefully monitored after traumatic events.

> *Key Point*: Anxiety *symptoms* may resolve as part of the standard treatment of bipolar disorder, but anxiety *disorders* need to be managed as second conditions, with an eye toward integrated treatment whenever possible.

4.2.5. Attention Deficit Hyperactivity Disorder

Co-occurring attention deficit hyperactivity disorder (ADHD) affects one-third of adults with bipolar disorder and up to 80% of bipolar children and adolescents. The decrease with aging in rates of co-occurring ADHD may be due to ADHD symptoms resolving over time. Alternatively, this decline in rates with age may represent a complex interplay between cognitive and brain development, genetic risks for bipolar disorder, and variable expression of symptoms as the illnesses progress. Consequently, several hypotheses have been proposed for the high rates of ADHD in bipolar disorder.[7]

Table 4.2 WHO Rates of Anxiety Disorders in Bipolar Disorder		
Condition	**Bipolar I Disorder**	**Bipolar II Disorder**
Panic disorder	18%	17%
OCD	18%	12%
PTSD	26%	25%
GAD	27%	33%
Social Phobia	35%	36%

WHO = World Health Organization; OCD = obsessive-compulsive disorder; PTSD = post-traumatic stress disorder; GAD = generalized anxiety disorder
Source: Adapted from Merikangas et al., 2011.[5]

1. Symptoms common to both conditions (e.g., inattention, impulsivity) lead to overdiagnosis of ADHD in bipolar individuals, particularly in children;
2. ADHD and bipolar disorder share risk factors; or
3. ADHD is a prodromal expression of bipolar disorder.

Research supports these hypotheses to some extent, although perhaps the best evidence suggests that ADHD is an early expression of an evolving bipolar illness in children before they develop mania. As illness progresses, these ADHD symptoms become more clearly components of affective episodes, leading to decreases in the rates of this co-occurrence over time. Regardless, ADHD in a child with familial risk for bipolar disorder suggests increased diligence during treatment and follow-up for the emergence of depression and mania. Indeed, stimulant exposure may precipitate mood symptoms in these at-risk children. Consequently, consideration should be given for alternative treatments for ADHD or concurrent prescribing of a mood stabilizer if mood symptoms are emerging in these at-risk kids; these considerations are discussed further in Chapter 8.

> *Key Point*: Clinical implications of co-occurring ADHD in bipolar disorder are dependent in part on the developmental stage of the individual.

4.2.6. Personality Disorders

The dynamic symptoms of bipolar disorder can be difficult to distinguish from the affective instability and cognitive symptoms of personality disorders, particularly those of DSM-5 cluster B disorders (e.g., borderline, histrionic, or narcissistic personality disorders). Consequently, a diagnosis of a co-occurring personality disorder demands ongoing behavioral characteristics that persist beyond mood states into euthymia. Recent studies that controlled for mood state in bipolar disorder still report high rates of co-occurring personality disorders.[8] Elevated rates of borderline, narcissistic, histrionic, obsessive-compulsive, and avoidant personality disorders are particularly common and occur in up to half of bipolar individuals. The presence of a personality disorder decreases treatment adherence, leads to lower rates of recovery, increases the risk of drug and alcohol abuse (further complicating course of illness), and increases the risk of suicide. Personality disorders typically require long-term and focused psychotherapies (e.g., dialectical behavioral therapy) to gain improvement, in addition to treating the primary bipolar disorder.

4.3. Co-occurring Medical Illnesses

Individuals with bipolar disorder have higher rates of medical illnesses and premature mortality due to these illnesses than the general population.[9] Attending to co-occurring medical illnesses, in general, is therefore an essential part of managing bipolar disorder. In addition to this general increased risk, there are several medical illnesses that are more common in bipolar

Table 4.3 Common Medical Conditions in Bipolar Disorder

Condition	Bipolar Disorder	General Population
Obesity	21–35%	20–36%
Diabetes (type II)	8–17%	6–8%
Cardiovascular disease	11–50%[1]	7–20%[1]
Migraine	25–40%	7–16%

[1] Widely variable depending on sample demographics

disorder than would be expected from general population prevalence rates. These are listed in Table 4.3 and discussed subsequently.

4.3.1. Metabolic Disorders/Diabetes/Overweight

The metabolic syndrome is a group of risk factors that increase the likelihood of heart disease, stroke, and diabetes; these risk factors are listed in Box 4.1. The metabolic syndrome is present in 30–50% of individuals with bipolar disorder, which is approximately a two-fold increase over the general population (although reported rates are widely variable). Particularly common are obesity and type II diabetes mellitus.[10,11]

High rates of overweight (BMI > 25) and obesity (BMI > 30) have been reported in multiple studies of individuals with bipolar disorder. Complicating interpretation, however, is a background in the United States of an overweight general population. Nonetheless, adjusting for dates of reports as well as age and other demographics, it appears that bipolar individuals may be at increased risk for obesity and overweight beginning at a younger age. Although often attributed to psychotropic medication exposure, which certainly is a contributing factor, high rates of overweight are observed even in treatment-naïve bipolar individuals. In this latter group, increased weight is typically associated with depressive episodes, suggesting a risk of obesity inherent in the illness. Notably, rates of obesity in bipolar disorder are higher in American than European samples, emphasizing the impact of general societal demographics.

Obesity is problematic for bipolar individuals as it represents a significant risk factor for other medical conditions including type II diabetes mellitus and

Box 4.1 American Heart Association Metabolic Syndrome—At Least Three of the Following

- Increased abdominal girth > 102 cm in men or 88 cm in women
- Elevated serum triglycerides > 150 mg/dL
- Low HDL < 40 mg/dL in men or 50 mg/dL in women
- Hypertension > 130 mm Hg systolic or 85 mm Hg diastolic blood pressure
- Elevated serum glucose > 100 mg/dL

Source: http://www.heart.org/HEARTORG/Conditions/ More/MetabolicSyndrome/ Symptoms-and -Diagnosis-of-Metabolic-Syndrome_UCM_ 301925_Article.jsp

the metabolic syndrome. Type II diabetes is up to three times more common in bipolar disorder than the general population, despite high rates of obesity in both groups. Consequently, other factors in the bipolar population may contribute to the elevated rate of type II diabetes. Specifically, type II diabetes has been associated with several medications used to treat bipolar disorder, especially atypical antipsychotics. Additionally, bipolar disorder may involve general hormonal dysregulation of multiple systems that include those responsible for glucose management. As noted, weight gain in bipolar samples may be shifted to younger age groups, thereby increasing the duration of overweight plus the interaction with developmental processes leading to type II diabetes.

4.3.2. Cardiovascular Disease

Cardiovascular disease is one of the two major causes of premature death in bipolar disorder that are increased compared with the general population (the other is suicide); bipolar individuals are two to three times more likely to die prematurely from heart disease compared with the general population.[9] Consistent with this statistic, the rate of these illnesses in bipolar individuals is two to three times higher than in the general population (Table 4.3). As noted previously in this chapter, individuals with bipolar disorder have a number of risk factors for cardiovascular disease that include high rates of obesity, type II diabetes, smoking, and drug and alcohol abuse. Conventional antipsychotics also add an additional risk of sudden death, and other medications commonly used in the treatment of bipolar disorder may add additional cardiac effects. Additionally, some studies suggested that even after controlling for these multiple risk factors, individuals with bipolar disorder may have an inherent increased risk of cardiovascular disease, perhaps related to hormonal dysregulation or inflammatory processes associated with bipolar illness. Given the risks, clinicians are encouraged to assist bipolar individuals in developing preventative health strategies (e.g., weight loss, stopping smoking) to prevent cardiovascular events.

> *Key Point*: Medical conditions related to the metabolic syndrome are particularly problematic in bipolar disorder. Specific attention toward cardiovascular disease is warranted as it is a leading cause of premature death in these individuals.

4.3.3. Migraine

It has been observed for decades, if not centuries, that individuals suffering from bipolar disorder also experience high rates of migraine. As noted in Table 4.3, nearly half of bipolar individuals develop migraines, and as many as two-thirds of women, which is three to six times more common than in the general population. In women, both mood symptoms and migraine may vary with the menstrual cycle. Migraine worsens the course of bipolar illness and is unfortunately often not addressed; many individuals with bipolar disorder and migraine never see a neurologist or other headache specialist. The specific cause of this co-occurrence is unknown, although it may be related to abnormal serotonergic neurotransmission or inflammatory processes.

4.4. General Principles for Managing Co-occurring Conditions

As noted, the presence of bipolar disorder does not protect individuals from other illnesses common in the general population. Moreover, bipolar disorder may increase the risk of some psychiatric and medical conditions. To date, no single treatments have been identified that improve both bipolar symptoms and these co-occurring illnesses; therefore, the recommended approach is to use best practices for both conditions when they co-occur while trying to minimize excessive medication prescribing. Treatment is discussed in more detail in Chapter 8.

> *Key Point*: Managing co-occurring illnesses in bipolar disorder typically requires concurrent administration and integration of best clinical practices for each condition.

References

1. Strakowski SM, DelBello MP. The co-occurrence of bipolar and substance use disorders. Clin Psychology Rev 2000; 20:191–206.

2. Regier DA, Farmer ME, Rae DS, Locke BZ, Keith SJ, Judd LL, Goodwin FK. Comorbidity of mental disorders with alcohol and other drug abuse. Results from the Epidemiologic Catchment Area (ECA) Study. JAMA 1990; 264:2511–2518.

3. Kessler RC, McGonagle KA, Zhao S, Nelson CB, Hughes M, Eshleman S, Wittchen HU, Kendler KS. Lifetime and 12-month prevalence of DSM-III-R psychiatric disorders in the United States. Results from the National Comorbidity Survey. Arch Gen Psychiatry 1994; 51:8–19.

4. Heffner JL, Strawn JR, DelBello MP, Strakowski SM, Anthenelli RM. The co-occurrence of cigarette smoking and bipolar disorder: phenomenology and treatment considerations. Bipolar Disord 2011; 13:439–453.

5. Merikangas KR, Jin R, He J-P, Kessler RC, Lee S, Sampson NA, Viana MC, Andrade LH, Hu C, Daram EG, Ladea M, Medina-Mora ME, Ono Y, Posada-Villa J, Sagar R, Wells JE, Zarkov Z. Prevalence and correlates of bipolar spectrum disorder in the World Mental Health Survey Initiative. Arch Gen Psychiatry 2011; 68:241–251.

6. Pollack MH, Simon NM, Fagiolini A, Pitman R, McNally RJ, Nierenberg AA, Miyahara S, Sachs GS, Perlman C, Ghaemi SN, Thase ME, Otto MW. Persistent posttraumatic stress disorder following September 11 in patients with bipolar disorder. J Clin Psychiatry 2006; 67:394–399.

7. Singh MK, DelBello MP, Kowatch RA, Strakowski SM. Co-occurrence of bipolar and attention-deficit hyperactivity disorders in children. Bipolar Disord 2006; 8:710–720.

8. Dunayevich E, Sax KW, Keck PE Jr., McElroy SL, Sorter MT, McConville BJ, Strakowski SM. Twelve-month outcome in bipolar patients with and without personality disorders. J Clin Psychiatry 2000; 61:134–139.

9. Roshanaei-Moghaddam B, Katon W. Premature mortality from general medical illnesses among persons with bipolar disorder: a review. Psychiatr Serv 2009; 60:147–156.

10. Calkin CV, Gardner DM, Ransom T, Alda M. The relationship between bipolar disorder and type 2 diabetes: more than just comorbid disorders. Ann Med 2013; 45:171–181.

11. Vancampfort D, Vansteelandt K, Correll CU, Mitchell AJ, De Herdt A, Sienaert P, Probst M, De Hert M. Metabolic syndrome and metabolic abnormalities in bipolar disorder: A meta-analysis of prevalence rates and moderators. Am J Psychiatry 2013; 170:265–274.

Chapter 5

Neurophysiology of Bipolar Disorder

5.1. Clinical Considerations

As discussed in Chapter 2, bipolar I disorder is defined by the occurrence of mania, whereas bipolar II disorder is characterized by hypomania plus at least one episode of depression. Both mania and hypomania are syndromes of extreme mood states, impaired cognition, neurovegetative symptoms and signs, and impulsive behaviors. Most bipolar individuals also experience recurrent depression with its additional mood, cognitive, neurovegetative, and other behavioral symptoms. Moreover, bipolar disorder commonly begins during adolescence and then exhibits progressive shortening of euthymic periods with increasingly frequent affective episodes. These clinical considerations suggest that neurophysiological models of bipolar disorder must describe a dynamic dysfunction of mood and cognitive brain systems beginning in adolescence that progresses over time to become a recurrent, life-long condition of diverse behavioral symptoms.

5.2. Emotional Brain Networks and Bipolar Disorder

Based on this brief review of clinical considerations, bipolar disorder appears to result from abnormalities in mood regulation. Like most complex human behaviors, emotional states are modulated by networks originating in the prefrontal cortex (see Figures 5.1 and 5.2).[1] The prefrontal cortex is a relatively complex, heterogeneous structure comprising multiple histologically distinct functional regions. Despite this complexity, each prefrontal region demonstrates a common architecture. Namely, each prefrontal area maps to specific corresponding regions of the striatum then thalamus then pallidum before connecting back to the originating prefrontal cortex to form iterative feedback and feedforward circuits (Figures 5.1 and 5.2). The various components of these networks receive sensory and other processed information from throughout the brain. From an evolutionary comparative anatomy perspective, as prefrontal cortical complexity increases, animal species demonstrate increasingly more nuanced variations of primitive "fight/flight" and reward-seeking behaviors; behaviors driven by the amygdala and ventral striatum, respectively.

Humans are distinguished from other animals by extreme prefrontal development that underlies the more subtle and complex emotional-social behaviors that characterize human interactions. Two prefrontal networks specifically modulate human emotional function, originating in the ventromedial and

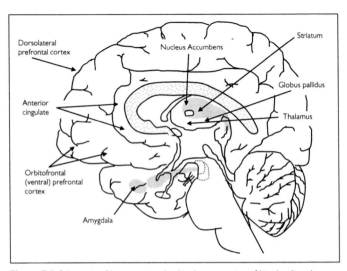

Figure 5.1 Schematic of key areas involved in the expression of bipolar disorder.

ventrolateral prefrontal cortices, respectively, and follow these same general patterns of organization as illustrated in Figure 5.2. The ventromedial prefrontal network processes internally referenced emotional states, that is, how a person "feels." The ventrolateral prefrontal network manages external emotional cues, for example, correctly interpreting facial expressions in others.

Although prefrontal networks are largely independent, they influence and inform each other through connections at various points along these circuits. Cognitive networks originate in dorsal prefrontal areas, but are reciprocally connected to emotional (ventral) networks within the anterior cingulate. Consequently, when ventral (emotional) prefrontal systems are activated, dorsal (cognitive) networks are deactivated; moreover, the converse also occurs. Consequently, primary dysfunction of emotional systems produces corresponding cognitive impairments; this model provides a framework for the functional neuroanatomy of bipolar disorder.[1]

> *Key Point*: Human emotional behavior is managed by two ventral pre-
> frontal cortical iterative networks that are reciprocally connected to
> dorsal (cognitive) networks. Together, dysfunction within these net-
> works likely underlies the symptoms of bipolar disorder.

5.3. Bipolar Disorder Results from Abnormalities in Emotional Networks

5.3.1. Amygdala

As noted, the amygdala is responsible for "fight or flight" behavioral responses to threats. In humans, ventral prefrontal networks nuance this response to

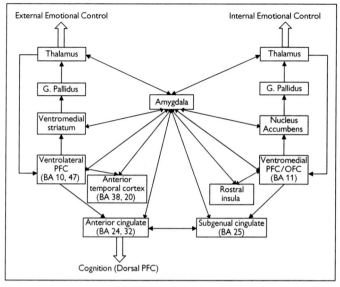

Figure 5.2 Schematic of the proposed ventrolateral and ventromedial prefrontal networks underlying human emotional brain networks (adapted from Strakowski[1]).

contribute to the wide range of human emotional states that characterize our species and that have gone awry in bipolar disorder. Consequently, given its central role in emotional behavior, the amygdala has been frequently studied in bipolar disorder.

One of the more replicable findings in psychiatry is that amygdala size in youth with bipolar disorder is decreased compared with healthy teens (Figure 5.3).[2] Moreover, we demonstrated that during the first year after a manic episode, bipolar adolescents failed to exhibit healthy amygdala growth, and, in fact appeared to experience amygdala volume loss compared with both healthy youth and teens with ADHD (Figure 5.4).[3] In contrast, a wide range of differences in amygdala volumes have been observed between bipolar and healthy adults, although perhaps most commonly, amygdala enlargement is observed in the former. This observation suggests that after amygdala underdevelopment in adolescence, there is a subsequent overgrowth of the structure in adults. This subsequent enlargement may be due to lithium or other medication exposure, however. Regardless, dynamic changes in amygdala structure and function appear to correspond with the progression of episode frequency that is observed clinically early in the course of illness (see Chapter 2).

Neuroimaging studies also consistently observe evidence of amygdala dysfunction that likely reflects these developmental anatomic anomalies. Perhaps most commonly, multiple studies across manic adults and adolescents report amygdala overactivation in response to facial affect. Amygdala overactivation has also been observed in healthy relatives of

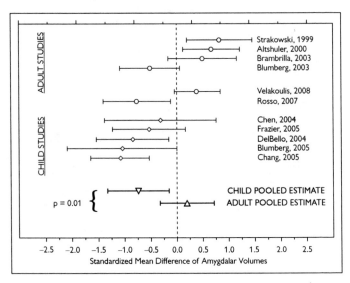

Figure 5.3 Studies of amygdala volumes in adolescents and adults—results of a meta-analysis (Pfeiffer et al.[2]).

bipolar individuals, suggesting that functional abnormalities may precede structural changes. In other types of cognitive tasks, amygdala underactivation is observed, suggesting a loss of healthy amygdala response specificity and flexibility to varying types of cognitive cues. During euthymia and depression, similar abnormalities of amygdala function are commonly reported.[1]

> *Key Point*: Bipolar disorder is characterized by loss of healthy amygdala function and flexibility in response to cognitive cues, reflected clinically in a loss of healthy modulation of emotional extremes.

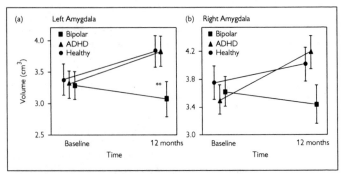

Figure 5.4 Trajectory of amygdala development in adolescents with bipolar disorder compared with healthy teens and teens with ADHD (Bitter et al.[3]).

5.3.2. Ventral Prefrontal Cortex

As noted, human emotion is managed by ventral prefrontal cortical networks. Not surprisingly, then, decreased activation in both lateral and medial ventral prefrontal cortical regions has been reported during mania, and to a lesser degree depression, across a wide variety of tasks. In contrast, during euthymia (remission), increased ventral prefrontal activation has been observed in the presence of amygdala overactivation (Figure 5.5).[4] This finding suggests that in this remitted phase of illness, underlying amygdala overactivation may be compensated by increased prefrontal control. Loss of this compensation, in response to stress or other factors, may then lead to mood episodes. In contrast to these findings in adults, in adolescents with bipolar disorder increased prefrontal activation is commonly observed. These observations suggest that, like amygdala abnormalities, prefrontal abnormalities in bipolar disorder develop over time. Finally, loss of prefrontal volume appears to occur with recurrent affective episodes and during the late teens and young adulthood. Indeed, adolescence is a period of significant changes in prefrontal cortical structure and function that appears to go awry in individuals at risk for bipolar disorder.

Supporting these considerations, neuroimaging studies commonly report abnormalities in functional connections between ventral prefrontal cortex and amygdala in bipolar disorder. During mania, functional connectivity is decreased between amygdala and lateral ventral prefrontal cortex that reverses with recovery (Figure 5.6). Similar, but more complex, functional disconnections occur during depression.

> *Key Point*: Mood episodes in bipolar disorder appear to reflect loss of ventral prefrontal modulation of the amygdala and other limbic brain structures.

5.3.3. Ventral Striatum

The ventral striatum includes the nucleus accumbens and ventral portions of the putamen and caudate that map to ventral prefrontal regions that comprise the

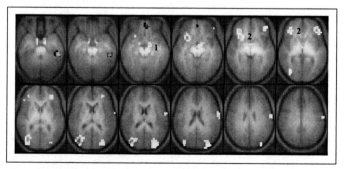

Figure 5.5 Ventrolateral hyperactivation in response to increased amygdala activation in euthymic bipolar disorder. Amygdala labeled with "1," ventrolateral prefrontal cortex labeled with "2." Dark colors indicate less activation in bipolar disorder; lighter (gray) colors are greater activation in bipolar disorder (Strakowski et al.[4] Reprinted with permission from Nature Publishing Group).

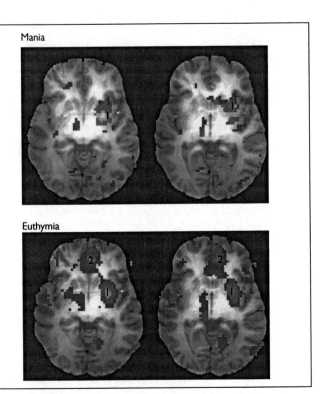

Mania

Euthymia

Figure 5.6 Changes in connectivity between right amygdala and prefrontal cortex during mania and after recovery (euthymia). Increasing brightness and extent of gray colors indicate increasing functional connectivity in prefrontal cortex (labeled "2") with right amygdala (labeled "1") (Cerullo M, Fleck DE, Eliassen J, Adler CM, DelBello MP, Strakowski SM, unpublished data).

emotional networks previously discussed. Closely linked to these structures is the globus pallidus. These brain regions receive extensive input from the amygdala as well as other brain areas, thereby providing an integrative role in emotion networks. As with other components of these networks, abnormalities in the striatum are commonly reported in bipolar disorder. Although some of these changes may be secondary to medication exposure, striatal and pallidal enlargement in bipolar compared with healthy subjects is observed in first-episode bipolar individuals and unaffected co-twins of bipolar probands. These findings suggest striatal abnormalities predate illness onset, prior to changes in prefrontal cortex and amygdala. Additionally, excessive striatal activation occurs in bipolar disorder, especially during mania. Disruption in function of these important integrative structures may consequently represent a risk factor for developing bipolar illness.

5.3.4. White Matter Findings: Abnormalities in Connections

Recent advances in MRI (e.g., diffusion tensor imaging) provide measures of white matter tracts. Using these methods, studies observed white matter abnormalities in ventral prefrontal and periventricular regions in bipolar disorder, consistent with loss of connections among the prefrontal cortex, striatum and amygdala; these findings are likely related to the functional connectivity abnormalities noted earlier. Studies of white matter in subjects at risk for bipolar disorder (i.e., that have a parent with bipolar disorder) suggest that these abnormalities predate illness onset. These premorbid white matter abnormalities may disrupt healthy developmental connections among ventral prefrontal networks and the amygdala, thereby setting a substrate that progresses to the first manic episode and a bipolar course of illness.[1]

5.3.5. Functional Neuroanatomy of Bipolar Disorder: Summary

When considered together, neuroimaging studies suggest that the symptoms of bipolar disorder arise from a loss of prefrontal modulation of amygdala and other emotional brain regions. This dysfunction is reflected in abnormal responses to cognitive cues of components of human brain networks that modulate emotion. This abnormal function is reflected in structural abnormalities in these same brain areas. These abnormalities appear to occur developmentally during adolescence, and as they evolve they lead to mania or hypomania followed by a progressive recurrence of mood episodes that defines a lifelong bipolar illness.[1]

> Key Point: Bipolar disorder is a developmental illness characterized by functional and structural abnormalities within prefrontal cortical brain networks that modulate human emotional behaviors.

5.4. Brain Metabolism and Bipolar Disorder

Magnetic resonance spectroscopy (MRS) provides techniques for studying the molecular substrate of the brain in vivo in humans and so has been applied to the study of bipolar disorder. The most widely used MRS technique measures hydrogen concentrations in various molecules. Using this technique (H1-MRS) neurochemicals studied in bipolar disorder include: n-acetyl-aspartate (NAA), choline, creatine, myo-inositol, and Glx. Glx is a mixed measure that includes glutamate, GABA, and glutamine, although in prefrontal cortex, it is predominantly glutamate. An alternate MRS method, P31-MRS, is based on the concentration of phosphorus and measures molecules relevant to cellular energetics, such as adenosine triphosphate (ATP), creatine phosphate, and high-energy membrane metabolites, for example, phosphomonoesters (PME). Most of these molecules exhibit differences in concentrations between bipolar and healthy subjects (Table 5.1).[5]

In their extensive review, Stork and Renshaw[6] concluded that MRS findings in bipolar disorder converge to suggest that mitochondrial function is impaired. Specifically, the neuron's typical reliance on aerobic processes (namely, oxidative phosphorylation) shifts toward anaerobic processes (glycolysis) in the bipolar brain; this shift is reflected in increased lactate and glutamate levels (during mood episodes), a decrease in total energy production and substrate availability

Table 5.1 Summary of Findings in Bipolar Disorder Comparing Metabolite Concentrations in Different Mood States with Healthy Subjects

Metabolite	Mania	Depression	Euthymia
NAA	↓	↑	↓↑
Glx	↑	↑	↓↑
Cr		↑	↓↑
Cho	↑	↑	↑
mI	↑		↑
PCr	↓	↓	↓
PME	↑	↑	↓

Up arrow is increased; down arrow is decreased. (Adapted from Kim et al.[5])

(decreased PCr and NAA), and altered phospholipid metabolism (elevated Cho and decreased PME). The specific lesion is unclear, although genetic studies suggest that, in some families, bipolar disorder is maternally transmitted (N.B., mitochondrial genes all come from a person's mother). Moreover, some of these shifts may simply reflect regional hyperactivation in emotional brain networks in bipolar disorder, as discussed previously. Additionally, excessive glutamate may cause neuronal injury or death, contributing to structural changes in gray and white matter, for example, abnormalities in diffusion tensor imaging measures of white matter tracts or losses of prefrontal cortical volumes, thereby uniting the structural, chemical, and functional abnormalities observed. This model is illustrated in Figure 5.7.[1]

> *Key Point*: Bipolar disorder is characterized by neurochemical findings consistent with abnormalities in brain energetics and mitochondrial function.

5.5. Neurotransmitter Hypotheses of Bipolar Disorder

5.5.1. Monoamines: Serotonin, Norepinephrine, and Dopamine

For decades, investigators hypothesized that abnormalities in the function of monoamine neurotransmitters, namely, serotonin (5-hydroxytryptomine; 5-HT), dopamine, and norepinephrine, caused affective disorders. These hypotheses largely arose from the neurochemical effects of antidepressants and, to a lesser degree, lithium and antipsychotics. Specifically, most antidepressants increase the availability of serotonin or norepinephrine (or both) in the synapse. Antidepressants may also increase the risk of a switch into mania when used in individuals with bipolar disorder (see Chapter 7). Additionally, antipsychotics block dopamine neurotransmission and are effective antimanic agents. Lithium has a myriad of effects that include changes in brain serotonin and norepinephrine function. Although monoamines originate in circumscribed brain nuclei, they are distributed widely throughout the networks illustrated in Figures 5.2 and 5.7.[1,7]

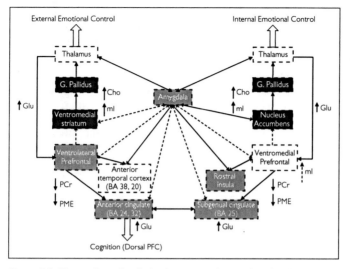

Figure 5.7 Abnormalities identified within emotional networks in bipolar disorder using magnetic resonance spectroscopy and structural and functional neuroimaging. Neurochemical abnormalities are noted with increased glutamate (Glu) observed in mania and depression throughout these networks. Increased *myo*-inositol (ml) and choline (Cho) are commonly observed across mood states in basal ganglia; increased ml (dotted arrow) is observed in orbitofrontal cortex prior to illness onset, in at-risk offspring of bipolar parents. Finally, prefrontal phosphocreatine (PCr) and phospholipid (PME) levels are also decreased. Other characteristics of the figure from structural and functional imaging are as follows: dashed border = brain regions exhibiting relatively consistent functional differences between bipolar and healthy subjects; gray boxes = regional structural abnormalities that appear to occur after illness onset (i.e., first manic episode); black boxes = regional structural abnormalities that may predate illness onset; dashed arrows = potential connectivity abnormalities identified in bipolar disorder using diffusion tensor imaging (adapted from Strakowski[1]).

5.5.1.1. Dopamine

Dopamine abnormalities in bipolar disorder have been relatively understudied, despite excess dopaminergic neurotransmission occurring in mania, as evidenced by the consistent finding that D2-receptor dopamine agonists (i.e., antipsychotics) are nearly universally effective antimanic treatments. Correspondingly, dopamine agonists such as amphetamine or L-dopa may produce manic-like syndromes. Brain dopamine is difficult to assay in human subjects, so that evidence of increased dopamine concentrations in bipolar disorder has been inconsistent. This inconsistency led some investigators to suggest that liability for mania may be related to supersensitive D2-dopamine receptors, rather than excessive dopamine *per se*; several studies suggested that lithium may prevent the development of dopamine receptor supersensitivity following antipsychotic administration. Moreover, gene studies reported findings in components of dopamine metabolism and function, including associations between bipolar disorder and D2- and D3-receptor alleles, dopamine transporter (DAT) genes, and catechol-O-methyl transferase (COMT) variants. COMT plays an important role in both dopamine and norepineph-rine metabolism. Lithium may alter dopaminergic activity within some brain regions, although this effect seems to vary with the timing and duration of treatment.[7]

5.5.1.2. Norepinephrine

Like dopamine, norepinephrine itself is difficult to directly study in humans. However, many antidepressants impact noradrenergic systems, and studies have largely established the occurrence of decreased noradrenergic neuro-transmission in major depression, independent of whether it is unipolar or bipolar. Additionally, some studies found relative increases in norepinephrine metabolites in mania relative to depression and euthymia, suggesting that increased noradrenergic neurotransmission and turnover may occur during mania. Gene studies reported associations between bipolar disorder and aspects of noradrenergic neurotransmission or metabolism including links with COMT (noted in the previous section) and tyrosine hydroxylase vari-ants. Studies of lithium and other mood stabilizers suggest complex associa-tions with noradrenergic activity that, like dopamine, appears to vary across brain regions and with the timing and duration of treatment.[7]

5.5.1.3. Serotonin and the Serotonin Permissive Hypothesis

Serotonergic abnormalities have been observed in studies of affec-tive disorders generally, although predominantly in subjects with unipo-lar depression. Findings include reduced serotonin metabolites (namely, 5-hydroxyindoleacetic acid; 5-HIAA) in the cerebrospinal fluid of suicidal indi-viduals; precipitation of depression with tryptophan depletion in individuals with histories of depression (tryptophan is a precursor of serotonin); and increased concentrations of serotonin receptors in mood disorders (mainly 5-HT$_2$). However, these findings have no specificity for bipolar disorder, but instead, and somewhat inconsistently, are associated with depression in gen-eral. More recently, a number of genetic studies observed abnormalities in serotonin transporter genes in bipolar disorder, although these findings have been difficult to replicate. However, 5-HIAA levels in cerebrospinal fluid may be reduced in both mania and depression, suggesting nonspecific changes with mood disturbances, rather than a direct relationship with bipolar disorder per se. Consistent with this suggestion, lithium both increases and decreases serotonergic activity; these effects depend on the brain region being studied and the duration and timing of lithium treatment, similar to norepinephrine and dopamine. Investigators interpreted these effects to suggest that lithium stabilizes monoamine function to lead to clinical improvement.

The actions of monoamines are not independent. Serotonergic func-tion is linked to activity in both noradrenergic and dopaminergic pathways. The findings of low serotonin levels in mood disorders in general coupled with changes observed during mania in the other two monoamines led to the "serotonin permissive hypothesis."[7] This hypothesis states that a pri-mary lesion producing low serotonergic tone results in dysregulation of both the dopaminergic and noradrenergic systems. Consequently, depending on other environmental and neural events, this low serotonergic function "per-mits" the release of dopaminergic and noradrenergic modulation leading to abnormal increases that produce mania and decreases that cause depression. This hypothesis has not withstood testing nor time, however, and many of these monoaminergic findings are now thought to represent epiphenomena of dysfunction in emotion networks, as well as abnormalities in cell signaling and mitochondrial function.

5.5.2. Glutamate and Gamma Aminobutyric Acid

Interest in the potential roles of gamma aminobutyric acid (GABA) and glutamate in the neurobiology of bipolar disorder arose from several considerations. GABA is the brain's primary inhibitory neurotransmitter and glutamate the primary excitatory neurotransmitter, so both are significant components of the communication pathways in networks that modulate emotion. Lithium and other mood stabilizers alter activity in both of these neurotransmitter systems. Moreover, as noted, MRS studies have relatively consistently observed increases in glutamate in bipolar mood states. Gene studies identified a few associations with genes related to GABA or glutamate activity. Unfortunately, studies of drugs with specific effects on glutamate receptors have not been particularly successful. Consequently the role of these two important neurotransmitters in the expression of bipolar disorder remains unclear, and, as with monoamines, abnormalities observed may simply reflect secondary findings from primary lesions elsewhere.[7] More research is needed.

> *Key Point:* Bipolar disorder is associated with metabolic and genetic abnormalities as well as treatment effects in the function of several major neurotransmitters, including dopamine, norepinephrine, serotonin, glutamate, and GABA. Direct evidence that these abnormalities are primary causes of bipolar disorder has been difficult to demonstrate.

5.6. Sleep and Circadian Rhythm Abnormalities

Sleep disturbances occur commonly in mood disorders. In bipolar disorder, mania is typically accompanied by disturbed sleep and, in particular, a decreased *need* for sleep. This latter symptom is unique to mania, although clinically distinguishing between decreased need for and inability to sleep can be difficult and these two experiences are not necessarily mutually exclusive. Moreover, studies suggest that mania and hypomania may be triggered by sleep deprivation in bipolar individuals; in fact, some have hypothesized that it is the sleep disturbance resulting from stress, rather than stress directly, that triggers affective episodes in bipolar disorder. As discussed in Chapter 7, protecting sleep is a critical part of a treatment program for bipolar disorder. Moreover, increased need for sleep, or hypersomnia, may be more common during bipolar than unipolar depression. Bipolar disorder may also demonstrate a seasonal pattern consistent with the lengthening and shortening of the day, namely mania in the spring and depression in the fall or winter.[8]

Together, these findings suggest that dysfunctional circadian rhythm regulators might underlie bipolar disorder. Several small studies found evidence of disrupted circadian rhythms in bipolar individuals that included a free-running "clock," phase-advanced or unstable rhythms, or loss of response or excessive sensitivity to environmental cues (zeitgebers). Unfortunately, replicating these findings in larger studies has been difficult. Additional evidence of circadian clock dysregulation was found in genetic studies in bipolar disorder in which abnormalities of clock genes were observed; again, these findings have been difficult to replicate.[8] Consequently, the specific causes of sleep disturbances in bipolar disorder remain unclear; however, management of sleep nonetheless appears to provide clinical benefit.

5.7. Cell Signaling and Calcium Metabolism in Bipolar Disorder

Studies of treatment response in mood disorders consistently raised the problem that many thymoleptic drugs (e.g., antidepressants) have immediate receptor binding and effects on monoamine systems, but clinical response is delayed by days or weeks. Moreover, mood stabilizers such as lithium have few direct cell receptor effects. These observations suggest that the neuropathology of bipolar disorder lies below simple receptor activity to cell signaling and epigenetic control. Moreover, as noted previously, MRS studies suggesting mitochondrial dysfunction in bipolar disorder are consistent with abnormalities in cellular metabolism and signaling. One mechanism that might explain these findings is impaired cellular calcium modulation. Impaired calcium metabolism is one of the most reproducible findings in bipolar disorder, and recent gene studies suggested that certain alleles of *CACNA1C*, a gene associated with cellular calcium regulatory processes, may confer risk of developing bipolar disorder. Moreover, as noted, MRS studies suggested that during mania and depression, glutamatergic neurotransmission is increased, and glutamate opens neuronal N-methyl-D-aspartate (NMDA) receptors leading to rapid calcium influx into cells and consequently into mitochondria. Too rapid an influx of calcium into mitochondria can disrupt production of ATP, the primary energetic molecule of the cell, particularly if mitochondrial metabolic processes are already inefficient. Impaired mitochondrial calcium regulation combined with increased glutamatergic neurotransmission within ventral prefrontal networks may therefore underlie the bioenergetic and hence functional imaging abnormalities observed in bipolar disorder.

Additionally, several of lithium's mechanisms of action impact calcium metabolism. Lithium is unique among psychotropic drugs in that it is relatively therapeutically specific, namely for the treatment of bipolar disorder, especially mania. Lithium inhibits inositol monophosphatase, thereby decreasing cellular inositol, which depletes phophatidylinositol-4,5-biphosphate (PIP2) and consequently inositol-1,4,5,-triphosphate (IP3). Since IP3 facilitates calcium release from endoplasmic reticulum stores, lowered levels of IP3 decrease the calcium burden on mitochondria, offsetting effects of excessive glutamate. This phosphoinositide signaling system also modulates protein kinase C (PKC) activity, which serves as a major component of cellular epigenetic and mitochondrial control.

Consequently, lithium effects mediated through inositol pathways might initiate a cascade of events leading to clinical improvement. Indeed, lithium also suppresses phosphorylation of the NMDA receptor NR2B subunit, thereby further modulating glutamate-induced calcium influx. It also increases bcl-2 (B-cell lymphoma-2 protein), which increases mitochondrial calcium capacity.

This latter observation hints at a mechanism for the previously discussed increases in gray matter associated with lithium administration; namely, that lithium is somehow neuroprotective. Indeed, bcl-2 modulates processes that protect against cell death (i.e., apoptosis). Lithium also inhibits glycogen synthase kinase-3 (GSK-3), a protein that sits within a number of intracellular signaling pathways that further protect again apoptosis. Modulated by monoamine neurotransmission, GSK-3 regulates circadian rhythm processes and impacts dozens of critical intracellular pathways. It is central to neuronal function and survival. Together these considerations suggest that lithium and perhaps other mood stabilizers and antidepressants correct a deficit in cellular signaling pathways that modulate neuronal energetics and plasticity as the primary lesion in bipolar disorder (see Schloesser et al.[9] or Goodwin and Jamison[7] for review). Additional work is needed to extend these observations.

> *Key Point*: Guided by the effects of lithium, studies suggest that bipolar disorder may arise from deficits in key cell metabolic processes and intracellular signaling that impact neural plasticity. Neuronal calcium handling may be central to these processes.

5.8. Summary of Bipolar Neurophysiology

From the considerations of this chapter, the model illustrated in Figure 5.7 was developed.[1] This integrated neurophysiological model of bipolar disorder arises from genetic variations in monoaminergic or glutamatergic regulation, mitochondrial function, cell signaling, brain development, and/or circadian rhythm regulation that disrupt the neurochemistry, structure, and function of emotional brain networks. Since the genetic etiology of bipolar disorder is likely heterogeneous, these genetic variations probably interact in several combinations, rather than all lesions occurring in all people, leading to dysfunction of emotional networks. Specific environmental events may be necessary to initiate epigenetic events leading to symptoms, although what these are remains essentially unknown. Regardless, abnormal development, bioenergetics, and modulation of these emotional networks appear to underlie emotional dysregulation and other symptoms of bipolar disorder, creating this complex, dynamic condition.

References

1. Strakowski SM. Chapter 13: Integration and consolidation: a neurophysiological model of bipolar disorder. In: Strakowski SM, ed., The Bipolar Brain: Integrating Neuroimaging and Genetics. New York: Oxford University Press 2012.

2. Pfeifer JC, Welge J, Strakowski SM, Adler CM, DelBello MP. Meta-analysis of amygdala volumes in children and adolescents with bipolar disorder. J Am Acad Child Adolesc Psychiatry 2008; 47:1289–1298.

3. Bitter SM, Mills NP, Adler CM, Strakowski SM, DelBello MP. Progression of amygdala volumetric abnormalities in adolescents after their first manic episode. J Am Acad Child Adolesc Psychiatry 2011; 50:1017–1026.

4. Strakowski SM, Adler CM, Holland SK, Mills N, DelBello MP. A preliminary FMRI study of sustained attention in euthymic, unmedicated bipolar disorder. Neuropsychopharmacology 2004; 29:1734–1740.

5. Kim JE, Lyoo IK, Renshaw PF. Chapter 4: Neurochemical and metabolic imaging in bipolar disorder. In: Strakowski SM, ed., The Bipolar Brain: Integrating Neuroimaging and Genetics. New York: Oxford University Press 2012.

6. Stork C, Renshaw PF. Mitochondrial dysfunction in bipolar disorder: evidence from magnetic resonance spectroscopy research. Mol Psychiatry 2005; 10:900–919.

7. Goodwin FK, Jamison KR. Chapter 14: Neurobiology. Manic-Depressive Illness. New York: Oxford University Press 2007.

8. Goodwin FK, Jamison KR. Chapter 16: Sleep and circadian rhythms. Manic-Depressive Illness. New York: Oxford University Press 2007.

9. Schloesser RJ, Huang J, Klein PS, Manji HK. Cellular plasticity cascades in the pathophysiology and treatment of bipolar disorder. Neuropsychopharmacology Reviews 2008; 33:110–133.

Chapter 6

Genetics of Bipolar Disorder

6.1. Bipolar Disorder Is Familial

Bipolar disorder runs in families. This fact has been recognized for at least 500 years, if not longer. It is unusual in clinical practice to encounter a bipolar individual with no family history of affective illness. Studies to clarify specific familial risks began in the early twentieth century and accumulated particularly toward the latter half of the century. These types of investigations—namely family studies, twin studies, and adoption studies—helped to establish the heritability of bipolar disorder and to define relative familial risks.[1,2]

6.1.1. Family Studies of Bipolar Disorders

Family studies typically start with an affected individual (the proband) and then identify relative rates of illness among family members. As described by Nurnberger,[1] these studies clarify the manner of inheritance of bipolar disorder by addressing three questions:

1. Are relatives of an individual with bipolar disorder at increased risk for the condition compared with relatives of people without bipolar disorder?
2. Do other disorders share a familial risk with bipolar disorder; that is, do other related conditions occur at elevated rates in families as well?
3. Can a specific mode of inheritance be identified?

As reviewed by Goodwin and Jamison,[2] family studies of bipolar disorder in general found that, on average, first-degree family members have a 12% rate of bipolar disorder, essentially a 10-fold increase over the general population. First-degree family members also exhibit a two-fold increased risk of unipolar major depression; in fact, due to its high prevalence, unipolar major depression is more common in bipolar families than bipolar disorder. Studies since approximately 1980 attempted to better delineate the relative risks in families of specific subtypes of bipolar disorder, namely types I and II. These results are summarized in Table 6.1. As illustrated, neither subtype of bipolar disorder "breeds true" in that both have increased rates of the other as well as of unipolar major depression; however, the relative risk of each type of mood disorder is increased based on the proband's subtype.

Unfortunately, the specific mode of inheritance of bipolar disorder remains unclear as it varies among different families from transmission that resembles strict Mendelian dominant or recessive patterns to maternal inheritance (as mentioned in Chapter 5). It is likely that this variability reflects multiple risk genes as discussed in section 6.2.2.

Table 6.1 Rates (Percentages) of Bipolar Disorders and Unipolar Major Depression from Family Studies

Proband	BPI	BPII	MDD
Bipolar I Disorder	5.2	3.8	16.6
Bipolar II	2.1	6.5	21.6
Major Depression	0.8	2.4	20.5
Healthy Population	0.1	0.9	7.3

Source: Adapted from Goodwin and Jamison[2]

6.1.2. Twin Studies

While bipolar disorder runs in families, this does not necessarily mean that it is genetic, since families share both genes and a common environment. Consequently, the environment could be the primary cause of this condition. Studies comparing monozygotic twins, who have 100% of their genes in common, with dizygotic twins, who share only 50% of their genes like any other siblings, provide one approach toward clarifying the relative contribution of genetics and environment. Specifically, if bipolar disorder is genetic it would be expected to more commonly affect both monozygotic (identical) twins than both dizygotic (fraternal) twins. Differences in concordance rates of bipolar disorder (between the two types of twins, i.e., rates in which both twins in a set are affected) can then be used to calculate a relative genetic risk for the condition. This relative risk is called the Holzinger heritability index (H^2),[1] and is calculated as:

$$H^2 = (monozygotic\ concordance - dizygotic\ concordance)/$$
$$(100\text{-}dizygotic\ concordance).$$

Although twin studies of bipolar disorder have been performed for more than a century with a wide variety of diagnostic criteria, the results are consistent. Namely, rates of bipolar disorder concordance are much higher in monozygotic than in dizygotic twins for both bipolar I and II disorder subtypes. For monozygotic twins, if one twin has bipolar disorder, the other has a 70–80% risk of developing bipolar disorder. For dizygotic twins, this risk is in the 15–25% range. Based on these differences, the heritability of bipolar disorder is 80–85%.[1-4] This genetic risk is higher than for any other psychiatric condition and most medical conditions. Nonetheless, since it is not 100%, some of the risk (15–20%) remains environmental. Environmental factors are not yet defined but could include significant neurobiological stresses such as trauma or substance abuse.

> *Key Point*: Bipolar disorder runs in families with 85% of the risk for developing this illness due to genetics. Nonetheless, the remaining risk likely reflects environmental factors.

6.1.3. Adoption Studies

An alternative approach to disentangle the relative contributions of genetic and environmental factors in the development of bipolar disorder is to use adoption studies. Adoption studies hypothesize that if the risk for bipolar disorder is primarily genetic, rather than environmental, then rates of bipolar disorder of children who are adopted will reflect that of the biological rather than adoptive parents. In bipolar disorder, these studies have typically involved identifying bipolar and healthy probands raised by either adoptive or biological parents and then examining rates of bipolar disorder in relatives of each combination. Few of these studies have been performed because they are difficult, but results have been consistent—namely that bipolar probands raised in adoptive families exhibit higher rates of bipolar disorder in the biological family of origin rather than the adoptive family. These results further support that the risk for developing bipolar disorder is primarily genetic.[1-3]

6.2. Genetics of Bipolar Disorder

The last two decades saw an explosion in methods to study the human genome, leading to increasing identification of genes that contribute to the development of human disease. Given its high heritability, bipolar disorder has been a consistent focus of these studies.

6.2.1. Linkage Studies

In humans, chromosomes exist in pairs, with one set of chromosomes, that is, half of the total complement of genes, inherited from each parent. Consequently, each gene is represented in duplicate; one member of each of these gene pairs is called an allele. During sperm and ovum formation, pairs of chromosomes separate in order to provide only one allele from each parent so that, when combined during fertilization, a full complement of genes is inherited. In the process of gamete formation as the chromosomes are separated (meiosis), genes "cross over" from one chromosome to another, thereby providing mixed combinations of genes from each of the grandparents. This *recombination* of genes is not random; genes farther apart are more likely to cross over (recombine) than genes that are close together. The latter, then are considered "linked" so that these copies of alleles are typically inherited together. It is this variability in recombination based on distances between genes that forms the basis of linkage studies.

Linkage studies measure differences in DNA markers (loci) located along chromosomes to identify whether specific loci are associated with the occurrence of bipolar disorder within families. The probability that a marker is linked to bipolar disorder is calculated as a logarithm of the odds of linkage or LOD score. Because it is logarithmic, a LOD score of 1.0 means that linkage is 10 times more likely than nonlinkage, for example. LOD scores greater than 3 are considered meaningful.

Early linkage studies raised considerable excitement by identifying potential genetic markers of bipolar disorder, but these findings proved to be difficult to replicate. Additionally, since a marker is not necessarily a gene, but is simply part of the chromosome near a gene that may be associated with bipolar disorder, linkage studies minimally advanced understanding of the genetic basis of the illness. Nonetheless, linkage studies identified markers associated with bipolar disorder on several chromosomes, with perhaps the best evidence for the short (q) arms of chromosomes 6, 8, 13, and 22, and the long (p) arm of chromosome 16.[1] These data provide additional evidence for the genetic basis of bipolar disorder, but have not identified specific genes that may be relevant. The occurrence of significant markers from multiple chromosomes was also an initial hint that bipolar disorder is polygenetic, that is, occurs from combined risks of multiple genes.

6.2.2. Association Studies

As noted, linkage studies define potential markers associated with bipolar disorder, but not specific genes. Association studies start by first identifying potentially relevant genes based either on the neurobiology of bipolar disorder or on linkage studies in which a promising gene is known to be close to a putative marker, and then evaluate whether the gene is associated with bipolar disorder. Often these studies use a proband and the two parents, called a trio, and then study multiple trios to determine the association of bipolar disorder with the gene of interest.

A more comprehensive set of methods, called genome-wide association studies (GWAS), were introduced in the past decade, becoming possible with advances in DNA chip technology in which millions of single nucleotide polymorphisms (SNP) can be evaluated in large samples all at once. Single nucleotide polymorphisms are small areas of DNA that show variability across human subjects in an otherwise relatively highly conserved DNA. Genome-wide association studies permit examination of virtually every gene in the genome, with the primary limitation being the statistical interpretation of thousands of data points. Consequently, to be effective, study samples must be very large, for example, in the tens of thousands. These methods have been applied to the study of psychiatric disorders in general and bipolar disorder specifically. As reported by Nurnberger,[1] several candidate genes potentially underlying the expression of bipolar disorder have been identified using these methods, and some of these have been replicated one or more times. None of these results has identified a specific cause of bipolar disorder, however. A few of the more promising findings are reviewed here and listed in Table 6.2.

D-Amino Acid Oxidase Activator (DAOA): DAOA function arises from two interacting genes (called *G30* and *G72*) that oxidize the putative neurotransmitter serine. Serine activates the N-methyl-D-aspartate (NMDA) glutamate receptor. Several clinical trials of serine have been performed in bipolar disorder, with inconsistent results. The gene is also associated with dendrite arborization, so may play a role in brain development.

Brain-Derived Neurotrophic Factor (BDNF): BDNF is a widely studied neuronal growth factor that plays a critical role in brain development and neurogenesis. Associations with different BDNF alleles have been found in a number of psychiatric and neurological diseases, including bipolar disorder.

Disrupted in Schizophrenia 1 (DISC1): DISC1 was originally isolated in a Scottish family with a genetic translocation and multiple cases of schizophrenia. Subsequent studies found that *DISC1* allelic variants were associated with other psychiatric conditions, including bipolar disorder. *DISC1* appears to control microtubule development in neurons, thereby contributing to brain development.

Table 6.2 Candidate Genes from Association Studies Potentially Involved in the Expression of Bipolar Disorder

Gene	Possible Function
DAOA	glutamate neurotransmission
BDNF	neurogenesis and brain development
DISC1	neuron microtubule formation
5HTT	serotonergic neurotransmission
COMT	monoamine metabolism
MAOA	monoamine metabolism
TPH1&2	serotonin synthesis
ANK3	impacts sodium channel structure
CACNA1C	calcium channel function
Source: Adapted from Nurnberger[1]	

Serotonin Transporter (5HTT): As discussed in Chapter 5, abnormalities in serotonergic neurotransmission have been frequently associated with major depression generally and, to a lesser extent, bipolar disorder.

Catechol-O-Methyl Transferase (COMT): COMT plays a significant role in the metabolism of dopamine and norepinephrine, both of which have shown abnormalities in bipolar disorder (Chapter 5). COMT allelic variants have been associated with a number of cognitive processes and across different psychiatric diagnoses, suggesting little specificity for bipolar disorder.

Monoamine Oxidase A (MAOA): MAOA metabolizes serotonin, dopamine, and norepinephrine, which all may play a role in the expression of bipolar disorder as noted.

Tryptophan Hydroxylase (TPH1 and 2): These two enzymes control the initial metabolism of tryptophan as a rate-limiting step in serotonin synthesis.

Ankyrin 3 (ANK3): This gene codes for a structural membrane protein involved in the formation of sodium channels. Sodium transport is central to the formation of neuronal action potential and, hence, neuronal communication.

CACNA1C: This calcium channel gene is associated with calcium function. As noted in Chapter 5, abnormalities in calcium metabolism are among the most common findings in bipolar disorder and also represent a potential mechanism of action for lithium.

As genetic technologies advance, it is likely that better understanding of these and other promising genes will arise. For example, sequencing studies using "next generation" methods (so-called next-gen sequencing) offer promise of more detailed analyses of the entire genome. Epigenetic research acknowledges that cells modify DNA transcription to impact the timing and expression of the underlying genome. The most commonly studied mechanisms to date are DNA methylation and chromatin remodeling. Neither of these methods has yet significantly impacted understanding of the genetic basis of bipolar disorder, but as the related basic neuroscience advances, we will be better positioned to understand results from older methods.

Key Point: Genetic methods have further established the genetic basis of bipolar disorder, but have not yet identified a specific gene or genes that cause the disorder. A number of promising candidate genes have been identified nonetheless.

6.3. Bipolar Endophenotypes

One of the major complexities associated with genetic studies of bipolar disorder is that, by its very nature, it is a behaviorally complex and dynamic condition. Consequently, identifying bipolar "cases" can be difficult, so at times studies have risen and fallen depending on the diagnoses of only a few individuals. To address this difficulty, recent efforts have attempted to identify endophenotypes to guide genetic studies. Endophenotypes are defined as biological characteristics that are stable, associated with an illness, directly measurable and, ideally, reflect known neurobiological processes. To date, endophenotypes have been difficult to define in bipolar disorder. However, one potentially useful endophenotype is lithium response, since lithium's therapeutic efficacy is relatively specific to bipolar disorder and, particularly, mania. Additionally, there is evidence that lithium response is familial and may be linked to chromosome 15q. Several large studies are underway using association methods to extend these findings.

6.4. Summary and Relevance for Genetic Counseling in Bipolar Disorder

Family, twin, adoption, and genetic studies provide overwhelming evidence that bipolar disorder is a genetic illness. Unfortunately, a specific "bipolar gene" has not been, and probably will not be, isolated. Instead, accumulating evidence suggests that bipolar disorder arises from the interactions among a variety of different genes that then interact with environmental stressors to precipitate illness. Moreover, it is similarly likely that different gene combinations interact in different families, complicating studies across groups.

Even in the absence of specific genetic tests for bipolar disorder, these studies provide guidance for family members of individuals with bipolar disorder. As illustrated in Table 6.3, the risk to an individual of developing

Table 6.3 Relative Familial Risks for Bipolar Disorder	
Situation	**Risk**
General population	1–2%
2nd-degree relative with BPD	3–4%
Sibling with BPD	15–25%
Parent with BPD	15–25%
Both parents with BPD	50%+
Identical twin with BD	70–80%

bipolar disorder increases with increasing genetic closeness and load within the family. However, the risk for onset is largely within the age range of 15 to 35 years, so risk decreases significantly in middle adulthood. Additionally, there is considerable variability among families, reflecting previous comments about the polygenetic nature of bipolar disorder. However, as genetic methods become increasingly powerful it is likely that these combinations will be increasingly understood, leading to meaningful developments in personalized treatment, disease prediction and, ideally, preventing the onset and progression of illness.[5]

> *Key Point*: Specific genetic tests are not yet available for bipolar disorder, although family history provides some information to counsel genetic risk within an individual.

References

1. Nurnberger JI Jr. Chapter 9: General genetics of bipolar disorder. In: Strakowski SM, ed., *The Bipolar Brain: Integrating Neuroimaging and Genetics*. New York: Oxford University Press, 2012.

2. Goodwin FK, Jamison KR. Chapter 13. Genetics. In: *Manic-Depressive Illness*. New York: Oxford University Press, 2007.

3. Bienvenu OJ, Davydow DS, Kendler KS. Psychiatric "diseases" versus behavioral disorders and degree of genetic influence. Psychol Med 2011; 41:33–40.

4. Bertelsen A, Harvald B, Hauge B. A Danish twin study of major affective disorders. Br J Psychiat 1977; 130:330–351.

5. Strakowski SM. Chapter 13: Integration and consolidation: a neurophysiological model of bipolar disorder. In: Strakowski SM, ed., *The Bipolar Brain: Integrating Neuroimaging and Genetics*. New York: Oxford University Press 2012.

Chapter 7

Psychopharmacologic Management of Bipolar Disorder

7.1. Introduction and Overview

As discussed in previous chapters, bipolar disorder is a complex, dynamic, behavioral condition. It should not be surprising, then, that treating bipolar disorder can be challenging and at times perplexing. However, by understanding treatment options and medical evidence, coupled with a programmatic approach toward maximizing psychosocial function, clinicians can help the vast majority of people with bipolar disorder lead successful and productive lives. In this chapter, we review evidence for pharmacologic treatments, placed within the context of often having to manage beyond strict evidence in given individuals. In Chapter 8, we will discuss psychotherapies and other treatments that complement psychopharmacology. Finally, in Chapter 9, we will pull everything together to conceptualize the treatment of bipolar disorder as a program, similar to other chronic, lifelong, and dynamic medical conditions (e.g., diabetes).

7.2. Psychopharmacology of Phases of Bipolar Disorder

Although the best treatment for bipolar disorder involves both medical and nonmedical components, effective psychopharmacology is required. For simplicity, pharmacological treatments are organized according to affective phase of illness, although this organization should not be interpreted to suggest disconnection of treatment across phases. The evidence base for drugs that are commonly used to treat bipolar disorder is listed in Table 7.1, with typical dosing ranges listed in Table 7.2. As illustrated, there are several potential treatment options for each phase of illness.

7.2.1. Treating Mania

As noted in Chapter 2, mania and hypomania are the defining syndromes for bipolar I and II disorders, respectively. Fortunately, the treatment of mania has been extensively studied, so that a number of USFDA-approved treatment options are available and, in general, most manic episodes can be successfully managed with one or more of these choices (Table 7.1).[1–3] When

Table 7.1 Commonly Used Pharmacologic Treatments in Bipolar Disorder, by Phase of Illness

Medication	Mania	Depression	Maintenance
Lithium	X	A	X
Conventional antipsychotics			
Chlorpromazine	X	D	D
Haloperidol	A	D	D
Atypical antipsychotics			
Risperidone	X	C	X[1]
Olanzapine	X	X[2]/B[3]	A
Ziprasidone	X	D	X[4]
Quetiapine	X	X	X[4]
Aripiprazole	X	D[5]	X
Lurisadone	C	X	C
Asenapine	X	C	D
Paliperidone	A	D	B
Clozapine	C	D	C
Antiepileptics			
Divalproex	X	B	B
Carbamazepine	X	C	B
Lamotrigine	D	A	X
Oxcarbazepine	C	C	D

Key: X = USFDA approved for this phase; if not USFDA approved then: A = replicated double-blind placebo-controlled clinical trial or meta-analysis demonstrating efficacy; B = at least one double-blind placebo controlled trial demonstrating efficacy; C = uncontrolled trials or expert clinical use/opinion; D = minimal evidence for efficacy or failed trials.
[1] USFDA approved in slow-release injectable form.
[2] USFDA in combination with fluoxetine.
[3] As monotherapy.
[4] USFDA approved for augmentation of lithium and divalproex.
[5] USFDA approved for augmentation therapy in major depressive disorder, not bipolar depression.

deciding where to place a drug in a treatment algorithm, evidence for efficacy as well as side-effect profiles and drug-drug interactions are considered. Moreover, whenever possible it is preferable to use antimanic treatments that can also serve as maintenance and antidepressant therapies, in order to simplify long-term management.

Table 7.3 classifies potential antimanic medications into first-, second- and third-line treatment options.[1-3] In general, all of the medications listed in Table 7.3 are similarly efficacious, in that approximately 50% of manic individuals will respond in 3–6 weeks on any one. One possible exception to this rule is that in so-called classic mania—early course, euphoric individuals—lithium exhibits response rates as high as 80%. Therefore, first-line treatments include drugs that are not only effective in mania, but also have efficacy in other aspects of bipolar disorder as listed in Table 7.1. First-line "1A" treatments include effective antimanic treatments that are typically USFDA approved

Table 7.2 Typical Dosage Range for Commonly Used Pharmacologic Treatments in Bipolar Disorder

Medication	Range (daily dose, mg)	Comments
Lithium	600-2400	Therapeutic range: 0.6-1.2 meq/L
Conventional antipsychotics		
Chlorpromazine	300-900	not recommended
Haloperidol	5-15	not recommended
Atypical antipsychotics		
Risperidone	2-6	slow-release injectable 12.5-50 mg q 2 weeks
Olanzapine	5-30	Fluoxetine combination available
Ziprasidone	40-160	not antidepressant
Quetiapine	200-800	mania dose higher (>500 mg)
Aripiprazole	5-20	only dopamine partial antagonist available
Lurisadone	20-160	not approved in mania
Paliperidone	3-12	IM dosing 39-234 mg monthly
Asenapine	10-20	sublingual administration
Clozapine	300-900	must monitor WBC levels
Antiepileptics		
Divalproex	500-2500	Therapeutic range: 50-150 mcg/ml
Carbamazepine	200-1600	Therapeutic range: 4-12 mcg/ml
Lamotrigine	100-300	not antimanic; slow titration required.
Oxcarbazepine	600-2400	limited data

but are downgraded slightly because of inadequate evidence for efficacy in other phases of illness, particularly relapse prevention. Of note, in children, lithium's efficacy is less well established, so it may be downgraded into this "1A" category as well. Similarly, due to its side-effect profile, some child psychiatrists would move olanzapine to "1A" or second line.

Despite its USFDA approval for the treatment of mania, the complex drug-drug interaction profile of carbamazepine lowers it to a second-line agent; it is also less well tolerated in general than other medications. Clozapine is an effective antimanic but has limited data in other phases of illness and a complex adverse-effect profile that places it as a third-line treatment. The conventional antipsychotics are less desirable due to extrapyramidal side effects, and they may worsen the long-term course of illness by inducing depression. Oxcarbazepine lacks sufficient data to move it higher. Electroconvulsive therapy (ECT) is an effective option in the treatment of mania, although it has been relatively little studied in this phase of illness. Nonetheless, in certain circumstances in which other treatments cannot be used, it is a reasonable choice.

A number of studies suggest that lithium or divalproex combined with an atypical antipsychotic may be more efficacious than lithium or divalproex alone in the treatment of mania. Not all combinations have been shown to

Table 7.3 Medications for Bipolar Mania
First-line treatments
Lithium*
Quetiapine*
Olanzapine*
Aripiprazole*
Risperidone*
First-line "1A" treatments
Divalproex*
Ziprasidone*
Asenapine*
Paliperidone
Second-line treatments
Carbamazepine*
Third-line treatments
Clozapine
Oxcarbazepine
Chlorpromazine*
Haloperidol
ECT
*USFDA approved

be better than monotherapy, but in general, these combinations appear to increase the rate of response to perhaps 60–70%.[3] However, some studies suggest that, rather than increasing the overall rate of response, combinations simply work faster than monotherapy. Regardless, in any given individual, the benefit of a more likely or more rapid response must be balanced against the greater risk for adverse events from adding a second medication.

The general pharmacological approach toward treating mania involves selecting a medication from Table 7.3 (or a combination of lithium or divalproex plus one of the atypical antipsychotics), starting at the lower end of the dosing range (Table 7.2) then titrating upward based on tolerability, treatment response, and, when indicated, serum drug levels. Typically, if an individual has responded to one of these drugs in the past, then it should be again chosen. If there is a history of a family member with bipolar disorder who responded favorably to a specific treatment, then that choice might serve as a starting point as well. Treatment response from any of these compounds occurs over a 3- to 6-week period, although many individuals will begin to respond within the first week. Additional details about each of these medications are provided later in this chapter.

Hypomania, as it occurs in both bipolar I and II disorders, follows a similar treatment approach. However, this milder phase of illness is commonly not reported by bipolar individuals, or may be managed by simply better maximizing the current relapse prevention therapy (discussed in section 7.2.4.).

Key Point: The treatment of bipolar mania has been well studied so that there are a number of USFDA-approved treatments that are similarly efficacious in mania. Choices among these drugs involve balancing any prior history of response and tolerability profiles.

7.2.2. Treating Depression

As noted in Chapter 2, although mania defines bipolar disorder, bipolar individuals struggle much more commonly with depression. Unfortunately, in contrast to mania, relatively few studies have identified effective bipolar antidepressants. At this time, only three compounds are USFDA-approved treatments for bipolar depression, namely quetiapine, lurisadone, and a combination drug containing fluoxetine and olanzapine (Table 7.1). Consequently, treatment of bipolar depression typically requires "off-label" use of medications that have demonstrated efficacy in studies (Table 7.1). First-line treatments for bipolar depression include the three USFDA-approved treatments plus lithium and lamotrigine (Table 7.4).[1,2,4] All of these drugs appear to be similarly effective such that approximately 50% of bipolar depressed individuals will improve in 6–8 weeks. Of note, however, negative clinical trials have been reported for both lithium and lamotrigine, both of which may be better for preventing depressive relapse than treating acute depressive symptoms *per se*. Lamotrigine treatment is further complicated by a very slow dose titration, making it less useful for severely depressed individuals in whom time may be critical. Lithium efficacy for bipolar depression in youth is not established. Again, these compounds are, in general, similarly tolerated as monotherapy.

Divalproex monotherapy is less consistently efficacious for bipolar depression in studies, and olanzapine monotherapy is less well studied (and perhaps tolerated), although both have antidepressant efficacy and other uses in bipolar disorder, leading to their second-line classification. The third-line treatments include compounds that either lack sufficient study or are less effective than the more highly rated compounds in Table 7.4. Several deserve comment.

Electroconvulsive therapy is an effective antidepressant for both unipolar and bipolar depression. For some individuals, it may be the best available choice and it may be considered first line in acutely psychotic, suicidal, or medically compromised individuals. Electroconvulsive therapy may also have a unique role in pregnancy (see Chapter 8). The role of standard (unipolar) antidepressants in bipolar depression is controversial. Although these drugs are widely used, recent large-scale, multisite studies suggest that they are ineffective in general for bipolar depression, although they may play a role in treating anxiety. Moreover, there may be a risk of precipitating mania or increasing the rate of mood cycling in some bipolar individuals; this risk appears to be highest for the older tricyclic antidepressants, which are, therefore, not recommended. When antidepressants are considered, they are best used in individuals already receiving effective relapse prevention therapy. Similarly, stimulants such as methylphenidate or dextroamphetamine may be useful in some depressed bipolar individuals, although the evidence base for this approach is underdeveloped. Like antidepressants, stimulants may increase the risk of mania. However, as noted in Chapter 4, more than half of youth with bipolar disorder experience co-occurring ADHD that may require a stimulant; in these cases, stimulants can be safely used as long as effective relapse prevention therapy is in place. Although not well studied, presumably this approach can also be applied to safely prescribe stimulants for bipolar depression in adults.

As with mania, there is some evidence that certain combinations may be more effective for treating bipolar depression than monotherapy. These combinations include lithium plus the newer antidepressants (e.g., SSRIs, bupropion), divalproex, or lamotrigine.[1,2,4]

The general pharmacological approach toward treating bipolar depression, then, involves selecting a medication from Table 7.4 or one of the combinations discussed previously and starting at the lower end of the dosing range (Table 7.2) then titrating upward based on tolerability, treatment response, and serum drug levels when indicated. Again, if an individual responded to one of these medications in the past, then it should again be chosen. Treatment response from any of these compounds tends to occur more slowly than with mania, often with little change during the first 1–2 weeks, and a full response may take as long as 8–12 weeks. Moreover, whereas mania often requires dosing at the higher end of the range, depression may respond at lower or mid-range doses. Additional details about each of these medications are provided later in this chapter.

This same approach is also reasonable for managing depression in bipolar II disorder, although there are relatively few clinical studies in this subtype. Unlike bipolar I disorder, antidepressant therapy may be more useful in

Table 7.4 Medications for Bipolar Depression
First-line treatments
Quetiapine*
Lurisadone*
Olanzapine/fluoxetine combination*
Lithium
Lamotrigine
Second-line treatments
Divalproex
Olanzapine (monotherapy)
Third-line treatments
Carbamazepine
Oxcarbazepine
Asenapine
Risperidone
Antidepressants (not tricyclics)
Stimulants (with established maintenance)
ECT
*USFDA approved

bipolar II disorder, perhaps even as monotherapy in those with predominantly depressive symptoms; however, more clinical research with this population is needed to identify more definitive approaches.

> *Key Point*: In contrast to bipolar mania, there are few USFDA-approved treatments for bipolar depression. Consequently, off-label treatments are often used. With few treatments and 50% response rates, more treatment options are desperately needed.

7.2.3. Treating Mixed States

In general, medications used for mania are effective in mixed states, although some are less effective in mixed than "pure" mania (e.g., lithium). When managing mixed states, therefore, mania recommendations should be followed.

7.2.4. Preventing Relapse: Maintenance Therapy

As noted throughout this book, bipolar disorder is a dynamic, complex behavioral disorder defined by mania, but characterized by manic, mixed, and depressive recurrences. Since functional recovery often trails symptom resolution by weeks or months following a major affective episode, preventing recurrences is critical for long-term good outcomes. Consequently, medications that prevent recurrences, namely, by increasing intervals between episodes, can have dramatic positive effects on outcomes. For most of the past 50 years, lithium was the only medication demonstrated to prevent affective episodes in bipolar disorder. Fortunately, during the past decade or so, a number of newer medications have been shown to be effective as well and have received USFDA approval for this indication; these are listed in Tables 7.1 and 7.5.

First-line maintenance therapies for bipolar disorder are listed in Table 7.5. Lithium has, by far, the most robust database supporting its use for relapse prevention not only from double-blind placebo controlled trials, but also from large scale, long-term follow-up studies of European lithium clinics. Lithium prevents both manic and depressive episodes and, perhaps uniquely, decreases suicidality. Lamotrigine appears to be primarily effective for preventing depression rather than mania. The atypical antipsychotics listed are typically more effective in preventing mania than depression, with the exceptions of quetiapine, which may be effective for preventing both acute phases of illness, and lurasidone, which has not established efficacy in mania.[1,2,5]

Divalproex is listed as second line because the one large-scale relapse prevention trial was negative; nonetheless, other trials and extensive clinical use suggest divalproex may be an effective maintenance therapy so therefore could be considered first line by reasonable clinicians. The other medications listed are promising, but lack data relative to first-line choices to move them to the higher category. Of note, when combined with lithium or divalproex, lamotrigine and these first- and second-line atypical antipsychotics further decrease recurrence rates compared with lithium or divalproex alone. The combination of lithium plus divalproex similarly may improve relapse risk compared with monotherapy of either medication. Again, the decision to combine medications involves a risk-versus-benefit analysis balancing the

Table 7.5 Medications for Relapse Prevention (Maintenance)
First-line treatments
Lithium*
Lamotrigine*
Aripiprazole*
Risperidone (long-acting injectable)*
Olanzapine
Quetiapine
Second-line treatments
Divalproex
Carbamazepine
Lurasidone
Paliperidone
Ziprasidone
Third-line treatments
Asenapine
Clozapine
Oxcarbazepine
*USFDA approved

potential decreases (typically of modest effect size) in recurrence rates against the increased likelihood of adverse events.

Third-line options lack sufficient data to recommend them more highly for relapse prevention. As noted previously, conventional antipsychotics appear to be ineffective for preventing depressive relapses and may even worsen the course of illness, so are not recommended as maintenance therapies. Similarly, the benefit of long-term antidepressant or stimulant use to prevent depressive relapses is not established.

Identifying the best maintenance medication is a long-term, trial-and-error process, and this approach is similar for both bipolar I and II disorders as well as other subtypes. As noted in Chapter 2, bipolar disorder is progressive, so that early in the course of illness, even untreated bipolar individuals may have several years between episodes. Even after progression stabilizes, affective episodes may occur at 12- to 18-month intervals, so determining the best prevention therapy often takes years of careful mood monitoring. Consequently, when treating acute affective episodes, it is best practice to start with medications that also have been demonstrated to prevent relapses (whenever possible), and then monitor the choice as an effective maintenance therapy over time. As will be discussed later in this chapter, a long-term treatment goal is to carefully monitor and record symptoms over time in order to identify the fewest medications necessary to get the maximal relapse prevention and tolerability. Although most bipolar individuals will require more than one medication for maximal relapse prevention, it is not recommended to prescribe more than three psychotropic medications unless clear circumstances necessitate such a choice. Indeed, there are no controlled studies of more than two concurrent medications in bipolar disorder. This number includes other ancillary treatments, such as hypnotics to help with sleep or benzodiazepines in the management of anxiety, so clinicians are advised to make wise medication choices based on careful long-term documentation of tolerability and treatment response. If an individual with bipolar disorder is on four different psychotropic medications and continues to be symptomatic, then it is best to reconsider all of the choices, pick the one or two that have been most effective, and start over with trial and error with alternative medications. Because bipolar individuals will therefore typically be faced with long-term medication therapy, tolerability becomes a major factor guiding treatment, and tolerability decreases with each medication added. Importantly, none of these treatments "cures" bipolar disorder; studies have shown that even after years or even decades of mood stability, most bipolar individuals will relapse within 6–12 months if maintenance therapy is discontinued.

> *Key Point*: Lithium remains the best-studied relapse prevention medication in bipolar disorder, although recent advances have increased treatment options. Often more than one medication is required to maximize outcome, but more than three medications is not recommended.

7.3. Specific Medications

7.3.1. Lithium

In 1946, Australian John Cade inadvertently discovered that, when injected into rats, lithium produced a calming effect. Subsequent studies in humans revealed that lithium was effective for treating mania. Concurrently, lithium was being used as a salt substitute and caused a number of deaths. These coincidental events highlight two important features of lithium: (1) is it an effective treatment for bipolar disorder; and (2) it has a narrow therapeutic window and can quickly become toxic. The toxicity effects delayed USFDA approval until 1970 (for mania), but in Europe, Australia, and elsewhere, extensive use and study of lithium identified it as the first efficacious, and relatively specific, treatment for bipolar disorder.

As noted, lithium is an effective antimanic, antidepressant, and relapse prevention treatment in bipolar disorder. Studies have shown lithium to be effective within 3–6 weeks in 50–60% of manic individuals, with tolerability, rather than inadequate efficacy, often being the reason for treatment failure. Side effects occur in more than 50% of treated individuals. In so-called classic mania, characterized by euphoria and minimal psychosis, the response rate of lithium is even higher, as much as 80%. In contrast, it is less effective in mixed states, and response rates in acute bipolar depression tend to be in the 40–50% range. Lithium is also more effective in individuals with fewer than 8–10 previous affective episodes, and its efficacy in children is unclear despite being USFDA approved in this age group. Notably, lithium is an effective antipsychotic in bipolar mania, equivalent to "primary" antipsychotics, despite having no efficacy in schizophrenia. Lithium significantly decreases the risk of manic and depressive relapses, and this improvement may accumulate over time.

Lithium is dosed to a therapeutic serum level, rather than only efficacy and tolerability, although typical dosages range from 600 mg to 2,400 mg per day. The therapeutic range for lithium is a trough level of 0.6–1.2 meq/L. Severe, particularly psychotic, mania often requires dosing at the higher end of the range, and there is still some controversy whether serum levels less than 0.8 meq/L are effective. Lithium is metabolized almost entirely by the kidneys, and studies suggest that it is excreted more rapidly during mania than during euthymia or depression; consequently the dose may need to be lowered as mania resolves in order to maintain a constant serum level. Because lithium has a serum half-life of 18–24 hours, steady-state serum levels are not achieved for 3–5 days, so that dosage adjustments are typically made on that schedule. Lithium can be administered effectively once daily, usually at night. In acute mania, lithium is typically started at 900–1,200 mg per day with dose increases occurring every 3–5 days depending on symptom response, tolerability, and serum levels. Titration can start lower and go a bit more slowly with bipolar depression, if necessary, to improve tolerance.

Initially, serum levels should be checked every 5–7 days to ensure serum concentrations within the therapeutic range; once the individual is stable, levels can be checked as infrequently at every 6–12 months. Because lithium requires serum levels and perhaps a bit more diligence in its initial management compared with other treatments (namely antipsychotics), it is now often disregarded in short-term, acute inpatient settings; this disregard is unfortunate, as lithium remains a first-line treatment for bipolar disorder (the author believes it is *the* first-line treatment); for many people, it is the most effective intervention. Although there are loading dose strategies that have been developed to predict the best "final" dose for lithium, these are rarely used because of toxicity concerns. Nonetheless, with experience, clinicians can learn to balance the pressures of short inpatient stays with the initial challenges of starting lithium.

Perhaps the limiting factor for using lithium is the risk of toxicity and side effects. Symptoms of toxicity include slurred speech, disorientation, ataxia, tremors, muscle twitches, cardiac arrhythmias, and nystagmus that can progress to coma and even death. Any significant acute lithium toxicity is a medical emergency requiring immediate attention that includes discontinuing lithium treatment, hydration, and aggressive supportive care. Nearly always, these symptoms resolve once the serum level returns to the therapeutic range.

Common side effects are listed in Table 7.6.[1] Gastrointestinal side effects are most common, but will often resolve over time; short-release formulations are more likely to cause nausea, whereas delayed-release preparations are more likely to cause diarrhea. Lithium is not typically sedating but does sometimes produce cognitive dulling that may not be tolerated; the latter may improve on lower serum levels. A mild tremor is common even on therapeutic doses (and sometimes a way to determine if someone is taking lithium even in the absence of a serum blood level). Lithium may cause acne, particularly in younger individuals. Weight gain, including an initial increase of 2–3 pounds of water retention, is relatively common, although not as significant as some of the atypical antipsychotics (e.g., olanzapine) or divalproex.

Table 7.6 Adverse Effects of Commonly Used Pharmacologic Treatments in Bipolar Disorder

Medication	Weight gain[a]	CNS[b]	EPS	Derm	GI	Comments
Lithium	++	+++	0	++	++	thyroid, renal, tremor; narrow therapeutic index
Conventional antipsychotics						
Chlorpromazine	+++	+++	++	+	++	anticholinergic, antihistaminic
Haloperidol	+	++	+++	+	+	tardive dyskinesia, hyperprolactinemia
Atypical antipsychotics						
Risperidone	++	+	++	+	+	hyperprolactinemia
Olanzapine	+++	+++	+	+	+	
Ziprasidone	+	+	++	+	+	QTc prolongation (clinically not significant typically)
Quetiapine	+++	+++	0	+	+	
Aripiprazole	+	+	+	+	+++	
Lurisadone	+	+	++	+	+	
Asenapine	++	++	++	+	+	
Paliperidone	++	+	++	+	+	
Clozapine	+++	+++	0	++	++	agranulocytosis
Antiepileptics						
Divalproex	++	++	0	+	++	polycystic ovarian syndrome
Carbamazepine	+	+++	0	+++	++	aplastic anemia, drug-drug interactions
Lamotrigine	+	+	0	+++	+	Stevens-Johnson syndrome
Oxcarbazepine	+	++	0	+	+	

Key: 0 = placebo rate or never; + = minimal or rare; ++ = moderate or occasional; +++ = severe or common.
[a]Also considers metabolic syndrome risk that often correlates with weight gain; [b]CNS includes sedation and cognitive effects.

Long-term use of lithium produces diabetes insipidus (i.e., increased thirst and urination) that results from changes in the ability of renal tubules to concentrate urine; this problem is not typically dangerous and usually is reversible, although can be bothersome particularly at night. Restricting water intake for the couple of hours before bedtime might help with nighttime awakening to go to the bathroom. Some studies suggest that long-term diabetes insipidus might lead to irreversible changes in renal function, probably in people with other risks for renal disease. Lithium inhibits thyroid hormone release, and chronic use may lead to clinical or subclinical hypothyroidism that requires hormone replacement. These renal and thyroid effects require laboratory monitoring (creatinine, TSH levels) that typically can be obtained concurrent with checking serum levels unless indicated earlier due to symptoms of renal or thyroid insufficiency. Evidence of abnormalities suggests a renal or thyroid work-up, respectively, is indicated.

7.3.2. Conventional Antipsychotics

At about the time lithium was being studied for mania, French physicians were using chlorpromazine as a pre-anesthetic and noted that it seemed to calm agitated patients. It was then tried in a group of agitated psychotic patients, who dramatically improved. Although in retrospect, many of these patients probably suffered from psychotic mania, the antipsychotic effects of chlorpromazine led to extensive testing in schizophrenia, thereby providing the first glimmer of hope for the treatment of one of humankind's most disabling illnesses. Eventually, chlorpromazine found its way back to the treatment of mania, in which it is also effective, and was USFDA approved for this use in 1973.

As discussed in Chapter 5, mania is a state of excessive dopaminergic neurotransmission, so that dopamine antagonists are essentially universally effective in its treatment. Although no other conventional antipsychotic has received USFDA approval for mania, there is convincing evidence that nearly all, if not all, conventional antipsychotics are effective antimanic treatments. For several decades, conventional antipsychotics, along with lithium, were the standard treatments for mania. However, as other drugs were identified, conventional antipsychotics fell into disfavor for bipolar disorder for two primary reasons. First, they impart a higher risk for the development of tardive dyskinesia and extrapyramidal side effects (EPS) than newer antipsychotics and may be less well tolerated in general (especially the low-potency antipsychotics like chlorpromazine). Second, conventional antipsychotics have not been found to be effective maintenance agents in bipolar disorder; in particular, they do not appear to prevent, and may even hasten, depressive recurrences. Nonetheless, these drugs remain third-line agents for acute mania in cases in which lithium, atypical antipsychotics or antiepileptics are either ineffective or not tolerated. Dosing for these compounds for the treatment of mania is typically the same as used for treating acute psychosis in schizophrenia. Although the rate and time course of treatment response is similar to lithium, the sedating effects particularly of low-potency antipsychotics are more pronounced and may therefore provide more rapid benefit for agitated patients earlier in treatment.

The side effects of representative conventional antipsychotics are listed in Table 7.6, although there is considerable variability depending on the relative potency of antidopaminergic versus anticholinergic and antihistaminic effects.[1] The primary concerns are with EPS, tardive dyskinesia, weight gain, and sexual dysfunction across most of these drugs.

7.3.3. Antiepileptics

In the 1970s investigators at the National Institute of Mental Health (NIMH) as well as several European centers began testing antiepileptics, primarily carbamazepine, in bipolar disorder based on hypothesized similarities in the clinical course of epilepsy (e.g., intermittent episodes, progression in symptoms) that were thought to potentially represent common underlying disease mechanisms. Although since then it seems less likely that bipolar and epileptic disorders share common etiopathological mechanisms, preliminary success with carbamazepine suggested alternative approaches to treating bipolar disorder.

7.3.3.1. Valproic Acid

Consequently, in the 1980s valproic acid was studied in mania and found to be effective; it was USFDA approved for this indication in the form of divalproex sodium in 1995, and it quickly became the most widely prescribed treatment for bipolar disorder for two primary reasons. First, divalproex has a much wider therapeutic range than lithium and is much less toxic at the high end of the range. Although formal serum-level-finding studies in bipolar disorder were never done, extrapolation from existing studies suggested that a serum level of 50–150 mcg/mL provides antimanic efficacy, although, again, some investigators prefer at least 80 mcg/mL or greater. Practically, given this wide therapeutic range, dosing is much more dependent on symptom improvement and tolerability than serum levels as compared with lithium. Second, pseudoloading dose strategies that predict a final steady-state dose in the therapeutic range were developed and well tolerated. Starting doses, then, of 20–25 mg/kg typically provide a good initial estimate of an effective divalproex dose. As with lithium, within 3–4 weeks, 50–60% of manic individuals respond to and tolerate divalproex. Serum levels should be checked every few days during initial titrations, but once response is established, these can be largely guided by clinical response and tolerability. Divalproex demonstrates less specificity, but broader efficacy than lithium, in that its response is similar independent of the presence of mixed states or multiple prior affective episodes. Its efficacy in bipolar depression is not well established. As noted, it did not separate from placebo on the primary maintenance study, although other studies and extensive clinical experience suggest divalproex has some relapse prevention qualities.

Although divalproex has a serum half-life of 9–16 hours, like lithium, it can be dosed once daily in bipolar disorder. Once the individual is stabilized, serum levels can be checked whenever performing routine follow-up of potential adverse effects of divalproex (Table 7.6). The common side-effects of divalproex include gastrointestinal (GI) disturbances, sedation, tremor, nonspecific pain complaints, and weight gain. Weight gain in particular can be quite significant (e.g., >25 pounds). In girls and young women, divalproex has been associated with increased rates of polycystic ovarian syndrome that can be significant and affect fertility; consequently, divalproex should be used carefully in these individuals and, when it is used, reproductive history should be monitored (e.g., menstrual cycle). Finally, rare but potentially dangerous side effects include hepatotoxicity, hemorrhagic pancreatitis, and thrombocytopenia. Consequently, hepatic profiles and blood counts are recommended perhaps annually or with symptoms; amylase should be checked with any significant abdominal symptoms.[1]

7.3.3.2. Carbamazepine

Although carbamazepine was studied prior to divalproex, it was not approved by the USFDA for the treatment of mania until 2004. The studies leading to this approval demonstrated antimanic efficacy that is similar in rates and timing of response to lithium and divalproex. The long delay in FDA approval occurred for several reasons. First, carbamazepine was generic, so there was little financial incentive to seek USFDA approval until a new delivery method was developed. Second, carbamazepine is relatively difficult to prescribe. Like lithium, it has a narrow therapeutic index with a serum concentration range of 4–12 mcg/mL. Third, carbamazepine has complex pharmacological properties. It induces the enzymes that metabolize it, leading not only to complex drug-drug interactions, but also to changes in its own serum levels over time. It can also decrease serum levels of oral contraceptives so that they become ineffective. Older studies suggest carbamazepine may be an effective antidepressant and may perhaps prevent relapse of affective episodes in bipolar disorders, although few, if any, of these studies would meet current double-blind, placebo-controlled design standards. Nonetheless, for the treatment of mania, carbamazepine is typically started at 200 mg twice per day then increased based on tolerability, clinical response, and serum levels. The typical dose range is 400–1,600 mg per day. As noted, serum-level monitoring can be useful to adjust dosing while awaiting a response (and avoiding side effects) and will need to be repeated for several weeks as carbamazepine autoinduces its own metabolism. Serum levels can be followed as other laboratory values are checked to monitor for adverse effects.

The common side effects of carbamazepine include GI effects, sedation, fatigue, dizziness, and dysphoria; many of these are dose dependent so improve with lowering the serum concentration (Table 7.6).[1] Carbamazepine may also produce a dose-dependent bradyarrhythmia. Up to 10% of individuals on carbamazepine develop a rash, of which a small percent progress to Stevens-Johnson syndrome, which can be life threatening. Occurrence of a rash, then, typically requires discontinuation of carbamazepine. Additionally, carbamazepine produces leukopenias in 7–10% of individuals with a 1 in 10,000 to 125,000 risk of aplastic anemia. Consequently, complete blood counts (CBC) including platelets should be checked every other week during the first 2–3 months of treatment and then whenever symptoms suggestive of leukopenia (e.g., fatigue, infection) occur. Carbamazepine also causes hyponatremia in 5–40% of individuals, so that serum electrolytes, particularly initially, should be followed along with the CBCs.

7.3.3.3. Lamotrigine

Lamotrigine is effective and USFDA approved for preventing depressive episodes and treating acute bipolar depression, although it has little, if any, antimanic efficacy. Consequently, it is commonly combined in the treatment of bipolar disorder with medications with the opposite profile (e.g., atypical antipsychotics, lithium, or divalproex). Lamotrigine is typically started at 25 mg per day for two weeks, then 50 mg per day for two weeks, then increased by 50 mg or 100 mg per week to the target dose of 200 mg per day (range 100–300 mg per day). Divalproex increases the serum levels of lamotrigine, requiring slower titration and a lower target dose when lamotrigine is added. Carbamazepine decreases lamotrigine serum levels, often requiring an increase in the dose of the latter when this combination is used. Oral contraceptives can also significantly decrease lamotrigine serum levels. This slow titration is believed to decrease the risk of Stevens-Johnson syndrome, the major side-effect concern with lamotrigine. Other common side effects include headaches, GI effects, or mild sedation. In general, lamotrigine is well tolerated in the absence of a rash.[1]

7.3.3.4. Other Antiepileptics

Several other antiepileptics are commonly used in bipolar disorder, but are not USFDA approved. Topiramate demonstrated initially promising results in small mania clinical trials, but then failed in large placebo-controlled studies in adults. In adolescents, one double-blind trial suggested that topiramate may be an effective antimanic in this younger age group, although the effect size was modest. Dosing for topiramate follows the titration used for epilepsy, namely starting at 50 mg per day and increasing by 50 mg per day each week until reaching a target dose of 100–400 mg based on tolerability and response. For children less than 10 years old, downward adjustments must be made based on weight. Common side effects include sedation, fatigue, paresthesias, and cognitive impairment, particularly word-finding difficulties. In particular, topiramate is associated with word-finding difficulties relatively unique to its administration. Unlike most bipolar treatments, topiramate is associated with weight loss rather than weight gain. It may cause nephrolithiasis.

Oxcarbazepine is chemically similar to carbamazepine, and several small clinical trials suggested that it is an effective antimanic, but data are limited. Serum levels for bipolar disorder are not known. Dosing is typically that used for epilepsy, namely starting with 600 mg per day and increasing up to 2,400 mg per day based on tolerability and response. Oxcarbazepine produces side effects similar to carbamazepine, although it tends to be better tolerated and the severe adverse effects (e.g., aplastic anemia, rash, hyponatremia) and enzymatic autoinduction are absent.

Gabapentin was widely prescribed for bipolar disorder for several years in the 1990s, until studies demonstrated it was no better (and perhaps even worse) than placebo in the treatment of bipolar mania. It has no role in the treatment of acute affective episodes or relapse prevention in bipolar disorder, although it may be an alternative anxiolytic to benzodiazepines or antidepressants for some individuals.

7.3.4. Atypical Antipsychotics

Although a specific definition of an "atypical" antipsychotic separating them from "conventional" antipsychotics has been somewhat elusive, the best functional definition is related to binding at the dopamine D2 receptor. Specifically, antipsychotic effects of these medications are thought to occur at D2 occupancy rates of about 65% with extrapyramidal symptoms (EPS) occurring at 85% occupancy. Conventional antipsychotic D2-receptor binding is such that the dose range between these two occupancy rates is very narrow and difficult to target clinically. In contrast, atypical antipsychotics either possess a larger dose range between these occupancy rates allowing more "targeted" dosing (e.g., risperidone), do not bind much more than 65% of D2 receptors at any dose (e.g., quetiapine) or are partial D2 agonists (e.g., aripiprazole). As a class, then, these drugs all bind D2 receptors, which likely accounts for antimanic efficacy, but have lower rates of EPS and tardive dys-kinesia than conventional antipsychotics. Moreover, unlike conventional anti-psychotics, some of these compounds appear to be effective at preventing and even treating bipolar depression.

As listed in Table 7.1, the atypical antipsychotics have, in general, all been demonstrated to be similarly effective antimanic agents, with response rates like lithium, and tolerability perhaps slightly better than lithium in the short term (weeks), although probably not in the long term (months); the excep-tion is lurisadone, which has not been studied in mania. These drugs do not require serum levels, but are dosed based on clinical response and tolera-bility; typical ranges are provided in Table 7.2. Despite variable half-lives, all can be dosed once daily, although sometimes multiple dosing is used to take advantage of "useful" side-effects, such as sedation in an agitated individual. In general, these drugs have been associated with weight gain and metabolic abnormalities, namely hyperlipidemia and type-2 diabetes. They also carry labels for potential risks for EPS, tardive dyskinesia and neuroleptic malignant syndrome, although specific risks appear to vary based largely on D2 dopa-mine receptor occupancy. Side effects profiles are listed in Table 7.6.[1]

7.3.4.1. Clozapine

Clozapine is the original atypical antipsychotic based on its D2 dopamine-binding properties. Although it represented a major advance in managing treatment-resistant schizophrenia, and it spawned the search for the next generation of antischizophrenia treatments, it is relatively uncom-monly used in bipolar disorder. Primarily, it is reserved for use in bipolar individuals with marked treatment resistance to other first- and second-line interventions. It has a complex side-effect profile that includes high rates of sedation, hypersalivation, tachycardia, dizziness, hypotension, and weight gain. Agranulocytosis occurs in perhaps 1% of individuals and can become life threatening; consequently, clozapine can only be prescribed within a specific registered program and requires weekly white blood cell counts (WBCs) for 6 months, then every 2 weeks for 6 months, followed by monthly checks from that point forward. Clozapine is typically started at 25 mg per day and increased by 25–50 mg per day to a target dose of 300–450 mg, based on tolerability and response. Higher doses may be used during acute mania.

7.3.4.2. Risperidone

Risperidone was USFDA approved for schizophrenia in 1993 and bipolar disorder in 2003; it also is approved for use in children and adolescents. Risperidone is an effective antimanic and maintenance treatment (primar-ily of manic relapse). Risperidone is typically started at 1–2 mg per day and dosed up to 6 mg per day (higher doses can be used, although tolerability decreases); in children, dosing above 3 mg per day is rarely indicated. The more common side effects include sedation, orthostatic hypotension, and dizziness. Risperidone is associated with weight gain, particularly in younger patients. It has a dose-dependent risk for EPS and akathisia and it can cause tardive dyskinesia. Finally, risperidone causes a dramatic increase in prolactin that may have long-term negative effects on reproductive functions and bone density.

7.3.4.3. Olanzapine

Olanzapine is an effective antimanic and maintenance agent and may be a weak antidepressant (which improves when combined with fluoxetine). It is USFDA approved for use in adolescents for the treatment of mania. In adults, it is typically started at 10 mg per day and can be increased to 30 mg per day; lower doses are commonly used in children. The most problematic adverse effects associated with olanzapine are sedation, which appears to persist throughout its treatment course, and weight gain. Indeed, olanzapine is associated with the highest weight-gain liability of any of these recommended treatments. It may also cause dry mouth and dizziness. The risk for EPS appears to be very low, at the level of placebo, and whether olanzapine causes tardive dyskinesia in bipolar disorder is unknown. However, it is associated with akathisia in general and with elevated liver function tests and prolactin in children.

7.3.4.4. Ziprasidone

Ziprasidone is an effective antimanic that may improve relapse prevention of lithium and divalproex when used in combination. It failed in bipolar depression studies, so is not recommended for the treatment of this phase of the illness. In mania, ziprasidone is typically initiated at 80 mg per day (40 mg bid) and titrated as tolerated and by response up to 160 mg per day. Ziprasidone is generally well tolerated, although it may cause dizziness or agitation. It is associated with QTc prolongation on the EKG, although this change has not had much clinical significance even with relatively widespread use. Nonetheless, it should be prescribed cautiously in people with personal or family histories of cardiac arrhythmias. It typically is not associated with significant weight gain. It may cause akathisia or EPS at higher doses. The risk of tardive dyskinesia is not known.

7.3.4.5. Quetiapine

Quetiapine is effective in all phases of bipolar disorder and is USFDA approved for use in children, teens, and adults. Quetiapine is typically started at 50–100 mg per day and increased based on efficacy and tolerability to up to 800 mg per day. Antidepressant and maintenance doses may be lower (e.g., 300 mg on average) than antimanic doses (e.g., 500 mg on average). The major side effects are sedation, which is often persistent, and weight gain. The latter can be significant (e.g., >25 pounds) and is particularly common in children. Quetiapine appears to have minimal or even no EPS liability, and perhaps a similar low or absent risk for tardive dyskinesia risk, consistent with its D2 dopamine receptor binding profile.

7.3.4.6. Aripiprazole

Aripiprazole is effective as an antimanic and maintenance agent (primarily for manic relapse) in bipolar disorder. It is approved for use in children and adolescents and is the only drug USFDA approved for maintenance treatment in this younger population. Although it has been USFDA approved for augmentation therapy in major depression, it has not demonstrated antidepressant efficacy in bipolar disorder. Aripiprazole is typically started at 5 mg per day (although it may be started even lower in children and individuals sensitive to side effects) and titrated within a few days to a target dose of 10 mg. Some individuals may require higher doses. The most common and problematic side effect for aripiprazole is nausea and vomiting, particularly initially. This side effect appears to diminish over time. Aripiprazole has relatively little weight-gain liability in adults, although is associated with weight gain in younger individuals. It can cause agitation or akathisia, although its risk for EPS and tardive dyskinesia appears to be low. Its use has been associated with an increased risk for stroke in elderly individuals with dementia.

7.3.4.7. Lurisadone

Lurisadone is an effective treatment for bipolar depression, but has not yet been studied as a maintenance agent or for mania. Given its efficacy in schizophrenia, however, it is likely an effective antimanic consistent with other dopamine antagonists. Lurisadone is typically initiated at 20 mg per day and increased based on clinical response and tolerability, perhaps as high as 160 mg per day. Lurisadone side effects include sedation, dose-related EPS and akathisia, GI disturbances, and a likely risk for tardive dyskinesia that is not well defined in bipolar disorder. It has relatively little association with weight gain.

7.3.4.8. Paliperidone

Paliperidone is effective as an antimanic agent and for prevention of mania relapse. It is USFDA approved for use in children and adolescents (for schizophrenia). Its efficacy in bipolar depression is not determined. Its side-effect profile is similar to that of risperidone, which is the parent drug (paliperidone is an active metabolite of risperidone). Paliperidone is typically started at 6 mg per day (corresponds to 3 mg per day of risperidone) and titrated to clinical response and tolerability. There is a long-acting injectable form of paliperidone that is started at 234 mg, with a second dose of 156 mg given one week later; then the typical monthly dose is 117 mg.

7.3.4.9. Asenapine

Asenapine is an effective antimanic agent, although it has not been established to be useful in other phases of bipolar disorder. It is administered sublingually and in mania typically started at 5 mg bid, then titrated to clinical response and tolerability. The common side effects include sedation, dizziness, dose-related EPS and akathisia, insomnia, and weight gain.

Atypical antipsychotics have significantly increased treatment options for bipolar disorder particularly for mania but more recently also for the treatment of bipolar depression and maintenance therapy. Choosing among them is generally based on efficacy across different phases (particularly in relapse prevention) and tolerability. Some of the newer medications are still under study so that additional trials may impact designations in Table 7.1.

> Key Point: Psychopharmacologic treatment options in bipolar disorder have significantly expanded during the past 20 years, allowing for many new possibilities and combinations. Clinicians are advised to familiarize themselves with all of these options, as they are all potentially useful within different clinical circumstances.

7.4. Conclusions

After decades of limited psychopharmacologic treatment options (namely lithium and conventional antipsychotics), during the last two decades there has been a dramatic increase in new medications to manage all phases of bipolar illness. Consequently, clinicians today have many more options than did their predecessors 20 years ago. Nonetheless, none of these medications is curative, and trial and error remains necessary to identify the best drug or drug combination for a given individual. In addition to new drug development, then, future research will focus on personalizing medication choices to maximize bipolar disorder outcomes. Medications are critical and necessary but not sufficient for best clinical outcomes, however, so additional therapies are necessary, as discussed in Chapter 8 and 9.

References

1. Strakowski SM, DelBello MP, Adler CM. Comparative efficacy and tolerability of drug treatments for bipolar disorder. CNS Drugs 2001; 15:701–718.

2. Yatham LN, Kennedy SH, Parikh SV, Schaffer A, Beaulieu S, Alda M, O'Donovan C, MacQueen G, McIntyre RS, Sharma V, Ravindran A, Young LT, Milev R, Bond DJ, Frey BN, Goldstein BI, Lafer B, Birmaher B, Ha K, Nolen WA, Berk M. Canadian Network for Mood and Anxiety Treatment (CANMAT) and International Society for Bipolar Disorder (ISBD) collaborative update of CANMAT guidelines for the management of patients with bipolar disorder: update 2013. Bipolar Disord 2013; 15:1–44.

3. Goodwin FK, Jamison KR. Chapter 18: Medical treatment of hypomania, mania and mixed states. *Manic-Depressive Illness.* New York: Oxford University Press, 2007.

4. Goodwin FK, Jamison KR. Chapter 19: Medical treatment of depression. *Manic-Depressive Illness.* New York: Oxford University Press, 2007.

5. Goodwin FK, Jamison KR. Chapter 20: Maintenance medical treatment. *Manic-Depressive Illness.* New York: Oxford University Press 2007.

Chapter 8

Psychotherapy and Complementary Treatments

8.1. Introduction

Although effective psychopharmacologic management is both necessary and critical to improve the course of bipolar disorder, it alone is typically not sufficient to maximize outcomes. In particular, research has shown that functional improvement often lags symptom resolution by weeks or months. Functional improvement is also only partially correlated with symptom resolution. Although medications contribute to functional recovery by decreasing affective symptoms, and perhaps by improving cognition, additional functional improvement typically requires psychotherapeutic interventions. The symptoms of affective episodes, for example, impulsivity in mania or the hopelessness and desperation of depression, often create significant psychosocial consequences, damaging interpersonal relationships, job performance, finances, and even enjoyment of recreation. Medications cannot address these issues. Certain psychotherapies may also be particularly useful for diminishing depressive symptoms as well as decreasing risk of relapse. Consequently, a comprehensive treatment of bipolar disorder requires use of evidenced-based psychotherapeutic interventions.[1]

8.1.1. Cognitive Behavioral Therapy

Cognitive behavioral therapies (CBT) are perhaps the most well established evidence-based psychotherapeutic treatments practiced in mental health care. As suggested by the name, CBT is based on two components. Originally developed by Aaron Beck, cognitive therapy works from the premise that depression (and other conditions) arises from negative automatic thoughts that are an individual's default response, setting them up for a vicious cycle of negative thoughts followed by corresponding negative behavior and expectations leading to additional negative thoughts that ultimately result in impaired function and behavioral symptoms (Figure 8.1). Cognitive therapy attempts to identify and modify these automatic negative thoughts to break the cycle. Behavioral therapy is an extension of this cognitive component in which modifications based on correcting negative behavior are implemented to further break this cycle. The reciprocal connections observed between the emotional and cognitive parts of the prefrontal cortex, as discussed in Chapter 5, provides neurobiological support for this basic premise that cognitive interventions can be used to modify emotional responses. Cognitive behavioral therapy has been shown to be

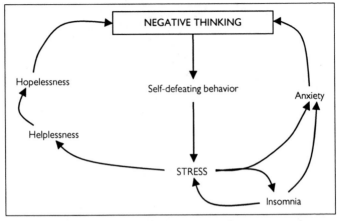

Figure 8.1 The vicious cycle of automatic negative thoughts.

effective in the treatment of depression, anxiety disorders, addictions, and a variety of psychiatric conditions. In many of these conditions, specific manuals have been developed and validated in clinical trials to direct the course of treatment. Cognitive behavioral therapy can be used both for the short-term management of acute symptom exacerbations and over the longer term to improve specific areas of function and cognitive approaches to life's stresses and problems.

Cognitive behavioral therapy has been less studied in bipolar disorder specifically than in other related conditions, namely major depression. In general, studies of CBT have been shown to improve recovery from acute depressive episodes and prevent affective relapses, although whether CBT is specifically superior to other psychotherapeutic interventions is not fully established.[1]

Box 8.1 Example Uses of CBT in Bipolar Disorder

1. Managing acute depression
2. Relapse prevention
3. Stress reduction
4. Interpersonal interactions
5. Medication adherence
6. Comorbidities
   - Anxiety and anxiety disorders
   - Alcohol and drug abuse
   - PTSD
   - OCD
   - ADHD
   - Eating disorders
   - Smoking

Regardless, given the efficacy in many other related and relevant conditions, the role of CBT in the management of bipolar disorder is likely to expand.

Currently, CBT has several important applications in the treatment of bipolar disorder (Box 8.1). As a well-established antidepressant therapy, CBT represents a first-line intervention for mild to moderate bipolar depression. In this role, CBT is used as an adjunct to existing maintenance psychopharmacology (e.g., lithium) instead of adding another medication. Cognitive behavioral therapy may also be a useful adjunct in nonpsychotic severe depression, although it may serve in a second-line role after additional psychopharmacology is initiated. The advantage of CBT over other interventions is that it has few adverse effects and does not interact with existing pharmacological regimens. Cognitive behavioral therapy has no demonstrated role in acute mania or in the presence of psychosis in any affective state.

In addition to its role in acute depression, CBT appears to improve relapse prevention when added to an existing maintenance medication regimen. Specifically, CBT can be applied to improve medication adherence, manage interepisode affective symptoms, and decrease stress by modifying maladaptive interpersonal and other behaviors. Additionally, evidence-based CBT approaches exist for many of the common comorbidities that occur in bipolar disorder including drug and alcohol abuse, anxiety disorders, eating disorders, PTSD, and OCD, as well as other conditions. Cognitive behavioral therapy, therefore, may be the treatment of choice for managing comorbidity, particularly when standard approaches to these conditions may be relatively problematic (e.g., antidepressants). Combined, these effects contribute to long-term functional improvement. Indeed, improvement from CBT may accumulate over time, presumably as individuals internalize more adaptive thought and behavior patterns. Moreover, when effectively administered, the additional cost of CBT appears to be offset by savings in other aspects of treatments management (e.g., fewer medications and hospitalizations). On balance, then, CBT is recommended for individuals with bipolar disorder.

8.1.2. Interpersonal and Social Rhythm Therapy

Interpersonal therapy has a long history of application in psychiatry and particularly in the management of depression. It operates from the premise that maladaptive social interactions are connected with depressive symptoms and so focuses on improving these interactions within the context of current relationships and symptoms, rather than past life experiences. No assumptions about causality or directionality are made. Ellen Frank and colleagues at the University of Pittsburgh advanced interpersonal therapy by focusing on social disruptions that immediately precede affective symptoms, thereby working from previous findings that interpersonal disruptions and the accompanying stress precipitate affective episodes.[2] As part of this therapy, it is postulated that a component of the risk for relapse derived from interpersonal stress is disruptions in social rhythms (e.g., sleep patterns) that interrupt the fragile circadian rhythmicity of bipolar disorder. Interpersonal and social rhythm therapy (IPSRT), then, focuses on first identifying maladaptive interpersonal behaviors and the disruptions in social rhythms that these cause. Once identified, the therapy moves toward reestablishing both healthy social rhythms (e.g., sleep, exercise, and eating patterns) in conjunction with managing interpersonal problem areas. Over time, the goal is for the bipolar individual to become independent of the therapist by learning to identify links among various social and biological components, developing more adaptive life strategies. Techniques from CBT are often integrated into IPSRT. Like CBT, IPSRT can be used both short- and long-term depending on treatment goals and each individual's ability to develop adaptive behaviors that can be independently maintained. Studies have shown that IPSRT enhances relapse prevention as an adjunct to medication. Whether it is superior to other therapies remains unclear, however.

8.1.3. Family-Focused Therapy

Family-focused therapy (FFT) works from the interpersonal model with the assumption that family members represent the most important relationships in the lives of individuals with bipolar disorder.[3] Unlike other interpersonal therapies, however, FFT works concurrently with both the affected individual and the family in order to identify and modify maladaptive interaction styles to improve communication, decrease individual and family stress, and advance all of the participants' understanding of bipolar disorder and its impact on family dynamics. Family-focused therapy acknowledges the stress and burden on the family members as they help manage bipolar disorder in their loved one. Family-focused therapy is also well positioned to manage the complex interactions in which multiple family members suffer from bipolar and other psychiatric illnesses, which, as noted in Chapter 6, is common in bipolar disorder.

Studies have found that FFT improves outcomes both in the short term during acute episodes and over time to prevent relapse. Family-focused therapy appears to increase medication adherence and decrease family "burn out." Family-focused therapy, then, is a useful adjunct to effective psychopharmacology, although it has not yet been demonstrated to be more effective than other evidence-based psychotherapies.

8.1.4. Education and Educational Therapy

The value to bipolar individuals and their families of understanding the course, expected outcomes, treatment options, and other aspects of bipolar disorder cannot be overstated. Education of individuals with bipolar disorder and their families improves outcomes by helping to better manage the illness by anticipating instead of simply reacting to symptoms. Education begins with talking to clinicians, but can rapidly expand to existing literature on bipolar disorder from national organizations such as the National Institute of Mental Health (NIMH) or the Depression and Bipolar Support Alliance (DBSA), from publishers, or from the Internet. Given the variability of material now available in an electronic world, it is recommended that treating clinicians guide individuals with bipolar disorder and their families to sites that rely on medical and scientific evidence to avoid misinformation. Education is really a lifelong venture and will need to remain an active part of any treatment plan and interaction throughout its course.

Additionally, recently Fristad and colleagues at the Ohio State University developed an educational approach that brings together parents of children with bipolar and other mood disorders to provide a group context and support for education.[4] This method, called multifamily psychoeducational psychotherapy (MFPEP) has been shown in studies to significantly improve outcomes in these children; it assists both parents and affected children develop skills in managing mood symptoms and the impact of those symptoms.

Box 8.2 lists common areas of education based largely on the outline of this book. Indeed, this book provides a starting point to guide clinicians toward potentially useful sources that can be adapted for individuals in treatment. It is recommended that clinicians develop a standard educational approach to apply within the context of their practice style, even when the focus is primarily psychopharmacology.

8.1.5. Supportive Therapy

Perhaps the most commonly applied therapy in clinical practice is typically a hodgepodge of education, encouragement, acute problem solving, medication management, and pieces from all of the previous discussed therapies that is referred to in combination as supportive therapy. Supportive therapy is inherently pragmatic and rarely structured. It can be (and is) delivered within the confines of even short medication visits. In research, supportive therapy is often used as a comparison treatment to structured therapies and at times it performs similarly. On balance, however, structured psychotherapies are probably superior, although clinicians to deliver these are not always available so that supportive therapy becomes the default. Consequently, it is recommended that clinicians familiarize themselves with structured psychotherapies and even if unable to follow them specifically due to time or resource constraints, nonetheless try to adapt key features into the supportive model to provide more consistent therapeutic interventions.

Box 8.2 Common Educational Topics in Bipolar Disorder

1. Clinical presentation
   - Symptoms
   - Diagnostic criteria
   - Early identification of relapse
   - Course of illness and prognosis
2. Common Comorbidities
3. Epidemiology
4. Neurobiology
5. Genetics and family risk patterns
6. Treatment options
   - Medications—risks versus benefits
   - Psychotherapy options
   - Lifestyle management
   - Treatment adherence
7. Finding a support group
8. Educational resources

8.1.6. Other Psychotherapies

Several other psychotherapies may be considered in the treatment of bipolar disorder. Dialectical behavioral therapy (DBT) is a manualized, modified CBT specifically designed to manage the suicidality and self-destructive behavior of individuals with borderline personality disorder. Dialectical behavioral therapy manages these behaviors by validating the associated thoughts and feelings while moving individuals toward more adaptive responses to them. Dialectical behavioral therapy has amassed a large database supporting its utility in borderline personality disorder in which it is the first-line intervention. Although not specifically demonstrated to be effective in bipolar disorder, given the relatively high rate of borderline personality traits in bipolar illness, DBT may be indicated for some individuals.

Psychodynamic psychotherapy has a long history in psychiatry, originally evolving from psychoanalytic roots. Psychodynamic psychotherapy works from an assumption that maladaptive behaviors are manifestations of subconscious drives and thoughts, often based on unhealthy upbringing. Some versions of psychodynamic psychotherapy, including strict, time-limited formats, have been demonstrated to be effective for depression. However, the evidence base for this treatment approach is minimal in bipolar disorder. Similarly, classic psychoanalytic psychotherapies using free association, dream interpretation, and other methods have not been demonstrated to improve the course or symptoms of bipolar disorder (or other major mental illnesses); consequently, at this time these therapies are not generally recommended.

> *Key Point*: Although psychotherapy is always used as an adjunct to psychopharmacology in bipolar disorder, several evidence-based approaches significantly improve overall treatment response and outcomes. Psychotherapies are almost certainly needed to maximally recover psychosocial function.

8.2. Complementary and Alternative Medicine in Bipolar Disorder

Complementary and alternative medicine (CAM) has become a catchphrase in modern medical practice as society struggles with chronic illnesses for which conventional medical treatments lack either sufficient efficacy or tolerability (or both). Although the boundaries between CAM and conventional medical practice are not always clear, generally CAM includes dietary supplements, lifestyle management, and non-Western traditional remedies. As noted earlier in this chapter, although effective evidence-based treatments for bipolar disorder are available, these often have significant side effects and typically only about half of individuals improve with a single intervention. Consequently, CAM is attractive to many individuals with bipolar disorder. Unfortunately, CAM approaches have not been adequately investigated in general for bipolar disorder, so that the evidence base is typically lacking. Nonetheless, a few approaches show promise.[5–7]

8.2.1. Dietary Supplements

Omega-3 fatty acids serve a variety of biological functions and cannot be synthesized intrinsically by humans, so we are dependent on obtaining them in our diets. Epidemiological evidence suggests that rates of depression may be higher in countries with lower dietary omega-3 fatty acids; these data in part led to a number of studies in major depression in which omega-3 fatty acid supplementation provided improvement. With these observations in mind, omega-3 fatty acids have been studied in bipolar disorder and appear to be effective for decreasing depressive symptoms in both adults and adolescents. To date, omega-3 fatty acids do not appear to be effective antimanic agents, and whether they prevent relapse is still unclear. Specific dosing of omega-3 fatty acids also remains undefined, but recent recommendations suggest starting with 1 g/day of a mix of eicosapentanoic acid (EPA) and docosa-hexaenoic acid (DHA) (i.e., the two subforms of omega-3 fatty acids) and then titrating upward based on tolerability perhaps to 3 g/day; however, of note, research studies raised the dose considerably further. Side effects tend to be dose related and are primarily gastrointestinal. Omega-3 fatty acids may also increase bleeding times at higher doses and should not be used in people with allergies to the source of the oil (e.g., fish).

Inositol has been examined in a number of studies primarily as an adjunctive treatment, because one of lithium's primary effects is to alter phosphoinositol metabolism (as noted in Chapter 5). Findings have been mixed. Because it is well tolerated, it is recommended by some guidelines as a third-line adjunctive option. Similarly, *N-acetyl cysteine* (NAC) was reported to improve depressive symptoms in bipolar disorder in one recent study, leading to its inclusion as a third-line adjunctive treatment. NAC is a precursor for glutathione, which is a brain antioxidant and so may improve inflammatory processes that have been proposed to be involved in the expression of bipolar disorder. However further investigation is needed for both of these treatments.

S-adenosylmethionine (SAM-e) is a cofactor in a number of biochemical pathways that may alter catecholamine function. This activity led to studies in depression with mixed results; to date, these studies have not supported its use in bipolar disorder. Similar observations have been noted for dietary tryptophan, a precursor of serotonin. St. John's Wort appears to have weak antidepressant properties, but it has not proven to be an effective or safe treatment for bipolar disorder. Melatonin has hypothetical interest in that it could be used to modulate circadian rhythms but, to date, has not been shown to be effective in bipolar disorder. However, for some individuals, it might provide an alternative to hypnotics (e.g., zolpidem) or benzodiazepines to help manage insomnia. Melatonin and melatonin-active compounds (e.g., agomelatine) may also improve mood symptoms, although studies are still preliminary. Finally, a number of preliminary studies examined supratherapeutic doses of a variety of vitamin supplements, but none yet have demonstrated efficacy.

8.2.2. Lifestyle Management

As noted previously, a key part of IPSRT involves modulating lifestyle behaviors, that is, social rhythms, to improve course of illness. Work with IPSRT supports interventions that help to stabilize sleep, eating, and exercise patterns. In particular, lifestyle techniques that manage and protect sleep appear to decrease the risk of affective relapse in bipolar disorder and improve overall course of illness. Direct benefits of regular, moderate levels of exercise have been examined in depression with mixed results; initially promising findings have been difficult to demonstrate in larger studies. Nonetheless, the general health benefits of regular, moderate exercise are well established. Drug and alcohol abuse, including cigarette smoking, have been demonstrated to worsen the course of bipolar illness, so lifestyle changes to eliminate these behaviors almost certainly improve outcome. Regardless of direct findings, healthy diet, exercise, and sleep patterns have substantial health benefits and so belong in the management of bipolar illness.

8.2.3. Traditional Therapies

Acupuncture has been a staple of non-Western medicine for millennia. Consequently, there have been recent efforts to determine its potential efficacy in depression and, by extension, bipolar disorder, primarily as an adjunctive therapy. To date, there is inadequate evidence to recommend this treatment for bipolar disorder. A variety of yoga therapies have been examined in psychiatric disorders, and yoga techniques are common mainstays for anxiety and stress management. In this role, then, they may have utility for individuals with bipolar disorder; however, there are no studies directly supporting yoga for managing primary bipolar symptoms. Again, although there is considerable enthusiasm for these treatments and risks appear to be low, benefits for bipolar disorder are not established.[5–7]

> *Key Point*: Although there is considerable enthusiasm for CAM in bipolar disorder, with the possible exception of adjunctive therapy with omega-3 fatty acids, evidence supporting these approaches is minimal. Nonetheless, healthy lifestyle management has multiple benefits to be recommended as part of bipolar disorder management.

8.3. Conclusions

Psychotherapies, particularly CBT, FFT, educational approaches, and IPSRT, have a key role in the treatment of bipolar disorder. Namely, psychotherapies complement psychopharmacology to maximize behavioral outcomes and function. A state-of-the-art programmatic approach to the management of bipolar disorder therefore requires the integration of psychotherapy with sophisticated psychopharmacology to maximize treatment benefit and outcome.

References

1. Goodwin FK, Jamison KR. Chapter 22: Psychotherapy. *Manic-Depressive Illness.* New York: Oxford University Press, 2007.

2. Frank E. *Treating Bipolar Disorder: A Clinician's Guide to Interpersonal and Social Rhythm Therapy.* New York: Guilford Press, 2005.

3. Miklowitz DJ. *Bipolar Disorder: A Family-Focused Treatment Approach.* New York: Guilford Press, 2008.

4. Fristad MA, Goldberg-Arnold JS, Gavazzi SM. Multifamily psychoeducation groups for families of children with bipolar disorder. Bipolar Disord 2002; 4:254–262.

5. Gracious BL, Gurumurthy S, Cottle A, McCabe T. Complementary and alternative medicine in child and adolescent bipolar disorder. In: SM Strakowski, CM Adler, MP DelBello, eds., *Progression of Bipolar Disorder in Youth: Presentation, Treatment, and Neurobiology.* New York: Oxford University Press, 2014.

6. Sarris J, Lake J, Hoenders R. Bipolar disorder and complementary medicine: current evidence, safety issues, and clinical considerations. J Altern Complement Med 2011; 17:881–890.

7. Ravindran AV, da Silva TL. Complementary and alternative therapies as add-on to pharmacotherapy for mood and anxiety disorders: a systematic review. J Affect Disord 2013; 150:707–719.

Chapter 9

A Programmatic Approach to Treatment

9.1. Introduction

As noted, bipolar disorder is a complex dynamic illness that impacts mood, cognition, and function across a wide range of behaviors and life spheres. This complexity requires carefully considered, thoughtful, and sophisticated treatment that integrates different modalities to maximally benefit affected individuals. Chapters 7 and 8 provide overviews of pharmacologic and therapy interventions, but to be most effective these must be built into a programmatic treatment approach to manage the range of behaviors and impairments associated with bipolar illness. This chapter develops an integrated program to guide treatment planning for people with bipolar disorder.

9.2. Pulling It All Together: The Program

Like other complex medical illnesses with dynamic courses (e.g., diabetes), optimal management requires more than simply prescribing a medication and sending people out to fend for themselves. Symptoms are multiple and changing and, by definition, cause marked psychosocial impairment. Functional recovery is often slow and is interrupted with every affective recurrence. Despite these challenges, most people with bipolar disorder lead relatively healthy lives, particularly with the right treatment program. These programs have several components, most of which we have already reviewed, that we will now put together (Box 9.1).

9.2.1. Comprehensive Clinical Assessments

Bipolar disorder (like all psychiatric and many other medical conditions) is a clinical diagnosis. There is no blood test or MRI scan that identifies the condition. Consequently, a comprehensive diagnostic assessment is the first step. To this end, each clinician needs to develop a semistructured approach toward initial psychiatric evaluations to be sure that a full psychiatric picture is obtained and to guard against prematurely jumping to diagnostic conclusions based on preconceptions or cultural biases. There are manualized approaches available, such as the Structured Clinical Interview for DSM-5 (SCID),[1] Schedule for Affective Disorders and Schizophrenia for School Age Children (K-SADS),[2] or the Diagnostic Interview for Genetics Studies (DIGS).[3] These manuals provide a process for obtaining consistent information from each individual. Although it is not necessary to use one of these interviews to

Box 9.1 Components of a Programmatic Treatment Plan

1. Comprehensive assessments
2. Ongoing safety evaluation
3. Aggressive management of symptoms and affective episodes
4. Building a support network
5. Set treatment goals—emphasize adherence
6. Integrate all aspects of care for long-term management in to a systematic appointment that:
   a. Evaluates primary and secondary (comorbid) symptoms.
   b. Reviews the mood chart.
   c. Reviews adherence to treatment.
   d. Reviews and supports general health measures.
   e. Performs safety assessments.
   f. Identifies new medical issues.
   g. Reviews drug and alcohol use, including smoking.
   h. Reviews and plans functional goals.
   i. Answers questions and provides education.
   j. Provides CBT or other therapy
   k. Makes treatment changes deliberately and systematically.

perform a comprehensive evaluation, the approach of following a specific process each and every time is a critical component of a comprehensive assessment. With this approach, it is often helpful to include specific symptom rating scales such as the Young Mania (YMRS)[4] or Montgomery-Asberg Depression (MADRS) Rating Scales[5] to assess the severity of symptoms and as measures to follow over time in order to interpret treatment effects. These and other rating scales are widely available online (e.g., YMRS at: http://psychology-tools.com/young-mania-rating-scale/; MADRS at: http://www.psy-world.com/madrs.htm). Importantly, these clinical assessments must include evaluations for conditions that commonly co-occur in bipolar disorder, as reviewed in Chapter 4.

Additionally, family history is a critical part of the evaluation; it is an unusual bipolar individual who does not have a family history of mood disorders, so this information can often guide both diagnosis and treatment decisions. However, because families often do not discuss mental illnesses, this information can be unreliable or spotty; in many cases, family history information does not come to light until after an individual has been in treatment for some time.

Ultimately, a major goal of treatment is to help bipolar individuals function as effectively as possible, even when managing mild to moderate symptoms. However, to identify realistic functional goals, assessments are necessary of prior ability to form relationships, employment history, educational achievement, and even recreational activities to guide functional goals later in treatment.

Consequently, diagnostic evaluations do not end after the first meeting; new information will become available during the course of treatment and with increasing collaboration between the clinician and the bipolar individual (and family members). Moreover, new medical and psychiatric conditions may develop during the course of illness that require treatment changes or alternatives, particularly in younger individuals. If treatment is not working as expected, the first assumption to challenge is that the diagnostic assessment was complete, so that ongoing reevaluation is the rule in bipolar disorder care (and mental health care more generally).

9.2.2. Ongoing Safety Evaluation

At times the major challenge in managing bipolar disorder is keeping affected individuals alive. The primary acute life-threatening risks in bipolar disorder are suicidality, psychosis, and impulsive and aggressive behaviors. Managing suicidality requires a careful assessment of potential risks in a given individual at a specific time and then making a thoughtful consideration of whether more restrictive care, including hospitalization, is required to keep the individual safe. Management of suicidal individuals is discussed in more detail in Chapter 10. Psychosis can occur in any mood state and, if sufficiently severe, can lead to impaired self-care or decision-making that may become life threatening. Similarly, impulsivity and aggression are common in mania and mixed states, and may lead to life-threatening poor decisions or harm to self and others. As with suicide, a careful risk assessment is necessary to determine the most appropriate level of care. As a general rule, when in doubt, err on the side of more restrictive care (e.g., hospitalization versus outpatient management).

In addition to these acute risks, commonly co-occurring substance use and medical disorders (e.g., cardiovascular disease) may become life threatening. Studies have shown that general practitioners often discount physical complaints from individuals with mental illness, so that psychiatrists will often, by necessity, need to assume a general medical role or help guide bipolar individuals to better medical care. Consequently, in bipolar individuals with medical illnesses, the treating psychiatrist and other mental health providers must remember to inquire about known medical conditions or new medical symptoms to provide this support. When a previously successful treatment regimen is suddenly failing, a high index of suspicion for these comorbidities may lead to a successful intervention prior to significant destabilization. New medical illnesses occur as a consequence of a recurrent illness, aging, and risks associated with high rates of obesity and smoking that occur in bipolar disorder. Managing these comorbidities is discussed in more detail in Chapter 10.

9.2.3. Aggressively Manage Acute Episodes and Interepisode Symptoms

Acute affective episodes can be life altering. In addition to increasing the risk of life-threatening behaviors, acute episodes disrupt psychosocial function in such a manner that can take weeks or even months to repair. The first step toward managing acute episodes is to prevent them. Careful review of common symptoms, particularly those that predict an ensuing full affective episode, must be part of every appointment. Once an episode occurs, the first step is to reevaluate the current treatment (if any) to identify whether it is really adding benefit or potentially contributing to the relapse (e.g., antidepressant therapy during a new manic episode), and to eliminate unnecessary interventions. The next step is to identify any possible triggers or precipitants (e.g., again, antidepressants during mania) and eliminate or modify them if possible. Then, appropriate alternative evidence-based management options, both medications and other therapies, are identified and deliberately and systematically initiated. Whenever possible, it is best to try to make one treatment change at a time in order to gauge the impact of that change; however, in severely ill individuals, this approach may not be possible. In these instances, once the patient is stabilized, critical review of the value of each treatment needs to occur.

Although acute episodes are the most destabilizing, significant symptoms that do not meet episode criteria also create significant morbidity. These symptoms not only include typical affective symptoms but also anxiety, which is associated with affective episode recurrence and poor outcomes. To manage anxiety, CBT is probably preferred, but benzodiazepines (in the short term) or serotonin-reuptake inhibiting antidepressants (in the longer term) may be useful adjuncts. Again, prevention is the better path when possible, but once these symptoms occur, deliberate, systematic treatment trials are indicated. Many treatments fail simply because of inadequate dosing or impatience, that is, not waiting long enough for the treatment to work. Both of these problems can be managed by clinicians sufficiently understanding the medications and therapies to appropriately prescribe them. Related, it is best to proactively manage symptoms by maximizing relapse prevention and monitoring for early indicators of recurrence, rather than reactively "chasing" symptoms. The latter strategy not only tends to fail but also often leads to intolerable and ineffective polypharmacy.

Because of the potential relationship between poorly modulated circadian rhythms in bipolar disorder and the onset of new affective episodes, a critical component of managing this illness is to protect regular sleep patterns. Developing approaches to healthy sleep hygiene is central to this process. Clinicians are advised to help bipolar individuals develop a predictable pattern of behaviors preparing them to sleep. When necessary, pharmacologic sleep aids such as hypnotics (e.g., zolpidem), benzodiazepines, low-dose trazodone (e.g., 50–100 mg) or sedating atypical antipsychotics may be useful additions toward this goal. When using these agents, a goal is to concurrently improve sleep hygiene so that medications are only necessary for short-term management.

In terms of providing medications, I recommend a treatment goal of three or fewer psychotropic medications at any time, as noted previously (Chapter 7). Although there are a few studies of combination therapy involving two drugs, there are none with three or more. If someone continues to have significant symptoms on three medications, then the medications are probably not offering benefit and so require reassessment and change. Again, changing one aspect of treatment at a time is preferred, remembering that bipolar disorder is a lifetime condition, so there is time for a deliberate, systematic intervention that is the best approach. A mantra I keep in mind is "We want to prescribe as much medication as needed but as little as possible."

9.2.4. Build a Support Network

Most individuals with bipolar disorder arrive at treatment for the first time with some psychosocial support, namely family and friends. Bipolar disorder can devastate relationships, however, so enlisting these important individuals in the person's care as soon as possible might create a more effective support system. Friends and family members can be enlisted to help bipolar individuals identify early warning symptoms to prevent episodes, manage the psychosocial consequences of affective episodes and symptoms, and aid with treatment adherence (particularly in younger individuals). Moreover, since bipolar disorder is strongly heritable, it is not uncommon for family members to be struggling with their own mental health concerns that may need to be coordinated to best support the entire family. A central component to building this support structure is regular education about the course of bipolar disorder in order to help set expectations and guide decision-making. As reviewed in Chapter 8, family-focused therapies can significantly assist with this process.

Bipolar disorder is a complex and at times mystifying and disabling condition that causes many affected individuals and their families to feel isolated, lost, and alone. Support groups help to combat these feelings by bringing together individuals with common experiences related to the illness in order to support each other, build a network of consumers of psychiatric and mental health services, and develop best personal practices to manage the disability of bipolar disorder. Because bipolar disorder is common, most communities have existing support groups. Often the best of these are linked to large national organizations that have developed a strong alliance with modern mental health care. The National Alliance for the Mentally Ill (NAMI)[6] and the Depression and Bipolar Support Alliance (DBSA)[7] are two national groups that have, over time, proven to be strong advocates and allies for people suffering from bipolar and related disorders and for their family members. Based on their national structure and size, these two groups have a number of helpful resources ranging from lists of local support groups to educational pamphlets and political action activities. They provide educational programs and drive community awareness to improve treatment of their members. Clinicians are encouraged to be familiar with these and other organizations in their area to guide individuals with bipolar disorder and their families. These groups provide a support network that is otherwise difficult to create, but that can provide real benefit to bipolar individuals and their loved ones. It is hard to overemphasize the importance of support group participation.

9.2.5. Set Treatment Goals: Emphasize Adherence

A major component of treatment success is to work with bipolar individuals to develop realistic treatment goals; overstated outcomes lead to discouragement, understated outcomes produce apathy. In order to set treatment goals, clinicians must take the time to understand how treatments work. For example, mood stabilizers typically produce side effects immediately, but treatment benefits trail by several weeks; initial improvement may not be evident for three weeks, and maximal benefit takes even longer. As noted earlier, there is some evidence that lithium benefits accumulate over months if not years, for example. A single session of psychotherapy is unlikely to be life altering. Consequently, as part of the educational process, it is recommended that clinicians set specific goals with individuals with bipolar disorder that integrate an understanding of evidence-based therapies and what the relative risks, benefits, and rates and timing of response are likely to be. These goals will ideally include not only symptom management, but also psychosocial functional improvement. The latter becomes increasingly important as bipolar individuals learn to distinguish normal moods from affective symptoms, understand the impact management of bipolar illness has on functional choices (e.g., whether or not to take a night-shift job), and learn how to integrate management of bipolar disorder into activities of daily living. Goal setting will evolve over time as individuals age and become more effective at managing their illness, so, like other aspects of bipolar disorder care, goal-setting is an ongoing process, not a one-time event.

A major goal for any treatment plan is to actually follow the plan. Nonadherence is a leading cause of treatment failure. Factors contributing to nonadherence are multiple and include poor insight into illness, lack of education regarding the need to follow treatment, insufficient support to help adhere to treatment plans, overly complex treatment (e.g., excessive polypharmacy) making it hard to manage, and a variety of cultural factors (e.g., the meaning of needing medication to different individuals). A first step toward managing treatment nonadherence is to develop rapport so that nonadherence will be reported and addressed nonjudgmentally. Mood charting (see section 9.2.6.) provides one method to monitor treatment adherence in which it can be somewhat impersonally recorded onto a chart, rather than having to face someone directly and admit it. Second, a well-developed educational program demonstrating the impact of not following treatment, repeated over time, may bring some individuals toward better adherence. Again, mood charting can be useful here, to demonstrate symptom emergence after not taking medication for several days, for example. Third, a well-designed CBT integrates treatment adherence of medication and therapy as part of the training, teaching individuals how to place treatment adherence into the larger context of cognitive restructuring leading to successful, healthy living. Finally, most people stop taking medications if the side effects outweigh the, essentially immediate, benefits (how many of you reading this book, for example, have actually completed every course of antibiotics?). Consequently, sensitivity to side effects in order to maximize tolerability can significantly enhance treatment adherence. This sensitivity requires clinicians to regularly inquire about side effects to be sure they are identified, reported, and addressed. For example, medications may contribute to sexual dysfunction, which is rarely reported if not directly asked about but is commonly a cause to stop treatment.

Ultimately, by virtue of its cyclicity, a major goal for bipolar disorder is to minimize affective recurrences and extend euthymic periods. This goal requires a long-term approach to this illness that requires both clinicians and bipolar individuals to develop specific habits that include regular monitoring of mood states and symptoms.

> *Key Point*: Thoughtful, realistic, and hopeful treatment goals are essential to guide treatment decisions and expectations. Managing expectations successfully can significantly improve treatment adherence and collaboration.

9.2.6. Mood Charting

As noted, bipolar disorder is a dynamic condition characterized by waxing and waning mood, cognitive, and behavioral symptoms and syndromes that may have variable and extended interepisode intervals. Even with effective treatment, symptom recurrences can and will occur. Moreover, since even evidence-based treatment relies on a certain amount of trial and error, identifying the treatment that is most effective for decreasing the numbers of episodes is challenging; therefore, it becomes critical to monitor changes in symptoms in response to changes in treatment over time. Unfortunately, in the absence of specific approaches toward making these measurements, both clinicians and bipolar individuals will rely on how the bipolar individual feels at the time of appointments, rather than reviewing course of illness over the previous appointment interval; this approach can be misleading as life events near the time of treatment (both positive and negative) can alter presentation in the short term that may be misattributed to treatment failure or success. For these reasons, daily mood charting is highly recommended. Even a simple record of mood symptoms or other individualized measures of treatment success (e.g., hours worked, decreased use of alcohol) help both the clinician and bipolar individual develop a process to monitor treatment over time. Ideally, the mood chart should record graphically to allow easy viewing and interpretation. Moreover, the charting can be extended and individualized to include potential mood triggers, such as hours of sleep, alcohol use, medication adherence, or stressful life events. Then, during appointments, weeks and even months of recordings can be reviewed to better identify the long-term effects of various treatment interventions. A sample mood chart is provided in the Appendix. Additionally, the technological (and especially cell phone) explosion has produced computer and phone programs and applications that can serve this same purpose (e.g., http://www.healthline.com/health-slideshow/top-iphone-android-apps-bipolar-disorder) and that may be more "user friendly." The key feature is to find a means of mood charting that is easy to complete, will be consistently used, and can be shared with clinicians to best manage mood cycling for a specific individual.

> *Key Point*: Bipolar is a dynamic, cycling illness managed through trial-and-error treatment assignment; consequently, mood charting is critical to determine the effectiveness of treatment interventions.

9.2.7. Integrate All Aspects of Care: Long-Term Management

Bipolar disorder, like other chronic recurrent, lifelong conditions, is managed rather than cured. To achieve this management, a long-term strategy is required; as noted, care needs to move away from reactive symptom "chasing" to proactive illness management. To do this, clinical care must be integrated across all of the dimensions reviewed. From the clinician side, this integration involves a multistep systematic standardized approach at each appointment that can be operationalized as follows:

1. Evaluate primary and secondary (comorbid) symptoms. Pay particular attention to and aggressively manage anxiety and sleep disturbances. Over time, work with the bipolar individual to define early symptom and behavioral symptoms of ensuing episodes, in order to intervene as soon as possible for prevention of episode recurrences.

2. Review the mood chart to identify symptom patterns over time and how symptoms respond to treatment interventions, in both the short and the long term.

3. Review adherence to treatment. Nonadherence to treatment is a primary cause of treatment failure. Building rapport to nonjudgmentally review adherence (e.g., recording on the mood chart) helps to identify the problem and develop educational or CBT-based interventions to improve adherence.

4. Review and support general health measures—for example, regular sleep and exercise. Help bipolar individuals develop healthy sleep hygiene and regular, predictable life rhythms.

5. Perform safety assessments of suicidal and other behaviors and thoughts as indicated. Hospitalization may be necessary to keep people safe in some instances. Work closely with each individual's support system to develop strategies for managing dangerousness.

6. Identify new medical issues and make medical assessments as indicated (e.g., weight, laboratory studies). Help bipolar individuals find internists and other specialists who do not simply dismiss physical complaints as part of the individual's mental illness.

7. Review drug and alcohol use, including smoking. Develop cessation plans.

8. Review psychosocial function and whether functional goals are being met.

9. Answer questions and provide education.

10. Provide CBT or other therapy with a focus on treatment adherence, managing interepisode symptoms (e.g., anxiety) and interpersonal behaviors, and decreasing the impact of life events (i.e., stress).

11. Plan treatment changes ideally one at a time. Make changes deliberately and systematically and monitor the impact of changes with mood charting.

Depending on the clinician's professional discipline, some of these steps make be distributed; for example, a psychiatrist might provide medical management and assessments in partnership with a therapist who provides CBT and setting functional goals. By providing systematic predictable care, clinicians can help bipolar individuals adopt corresponding deliberate habits in direct contrast to the dynamic sometimes chaotic course of bipolar illness; doing so will lead to best outcomes.

> *Key Point*: Due to its complex nature, bipolar disorder requires a deliberate systematic treatment program that addresses the broad nature of its expression.

References

Semi-Structured Diagnostic Interviews

1. First MB, Spitzer RL, Gibbon M, Williams JBW. *Structured Clinical Interview for DSM-IV Axis I Disorders- Patient Edition (SCID-I/P)*. Biometrics Research Department. New York State Psychiatric Institute, 722 West 168th Street, New York, NY 10032, 1995.

2. Geller B, Zimerman B, Williams M, Frazier J. *Washington University in St. Louis Kiddie and Young Adult Schedule for Affective Disorders and Schizophrenia (WASH-U-KSADS)*. St. Louis, MO: Washington University School of Medicine, 1996.

3. *Diagnostic Interview for Genetic Studies* v. 4.0. Rockville, MD: National Institute of Mental Health, 2004.

Symptom Rating Scales

4. Young RC, Biggs JT, Ziegler VE, Meyer DA. A rating scale for mania: reliability, validity and sensitivity. Br J Psychiatry 1978; 133:429–435.

5. Montgomery SA, Asberg M. A new depression scale designed to be sensitive to change. Br J Psychiatry 1979; 134:382–389.

Support Group Links

6. National Alliance on Mental Illness (NAMI): www.nami.org

7. Depression and Bipolar Support Alliance (DBSA): www.dbsalliance.org

Chapter 10

Managing Special Populations

10.1. Pediatric Bipolar Disorder

Most cases of bipolar disorder begin before age 21 years, so managing adolescents with bipolar disorder is common. Although differences between bipolar disorder in adults and youth are noted throughout this book, a few specific differences are highlighted here.

10.1.1. Diagnosis of Pediatric Bipolar Disorder

The diagnosis of bipolar disorder hinges on the occurrence of manic or hypomanic episodes. This requirement is the same in youth and generally applies well to older adolescents (e.g., >15 years). However, debate exists around diagnoses in younger children, in whom cognitive and emotional development can make "adult" symptoms of mania (e.g., grandiosity) difficult to interpret. In these younger groups, individuals meeting adult mania criteria are rare, yet research identifies a number of activated, irritable, and distractible children who may be expressing "atypical" bipolar disorder; these symptoms may also predict the onset of more "typical" symptoms in the future in these children.[1] Attempts to clarify the presentation of bipolar disorder in youth suggest that the strict episodic definition of mania used in adults may not represent the expression of bipolar disorder in children; namely, children may present with more chronic mood lability or irritability. Unfortunately, these symptoms occur in other common childhood conditions, for example, ADHD and pediatric depression.

Distinguishing ADHD from bipolar disorder in children is difficult. Perhaps the most useful approach is to focus on primary mood symptoms, especially euphoria, and evidence of episodicity, as these features are part of the course of bipolar disorder, but not of ADHD. A family history of bipolar disorder adds support for a bipolar disorder diagnosis. In many instances, the diagnosis may not be clear for months and may be informed by treatment response; for example, worsening symptoms with stimulant prescription might suggest bipolar disorder.

Pediatric depression is frequently expressed with irritability and agitation, making it difficult to distinguish from bipolar mixed states. Again, relying on the distinguishing features of mania (e.g., grandiosity, decreased *need* for sleep) along with family history data might clarify diagnosis. As with ADHD, a high index of suspicion while carefully monitoring treatment response may be informative.

Earlier onset bipolar disorder is associated with poorer long-term outcome and an increased genetic risk than typical onset. Given the complexities of diagnosis within the context of developing cognitive, emotional, and social neuropsychological functions, perhaps the best approach in youth is to maintain a

Table 10.1 Medications USFDA Approved for Treatment of Bipolar Disorder in Youth
For Mania
Lithium
Quetiapine
Olanzapine
Aripiprazole
Risperidone
For Maintenance
Aripiprazole

skeptical view of any initial diagnosis while gathering additional clinical data such as family history, symptom evolution, and treatment response.[1]

10.1.2. Treatment of Pediatric Bipolar Disorder

Although the treatment of pediatric bipolar disorder is similar in approach to that of adults, it cannot be assumed to be the same. Moreover, there are relatively few USFDA-approved medications for bipolar youth (Table 10.1). Notably, only the fluoxetine-olanzapine combination is USFDA approved for treating bipolar depression in children or adolescents, and no medication is approved below age 10 years.

Children and adolescents appear to be more sensitive than adults to many of the side effects of these medications. In particular, weight gain is much more problematic, even with drugs considered to be relatively "weight neutral" in adults. Consequently, attention to relative height and weight percentiles in individual growth curves must be followed carefully. Children and adolescents may also be more sensitive to cognitive side effects and so may benefit from lower doses to avoid excessive sedation or cognitive impairments. Conversely, young people typically metabolize drugs faster than adults, so that relatively higher doses (after adjusting for body weight) may be necessary; importantly, as children age, dose adjustments will be expected. Finally, prolactin increases occurring with some antipsychotics are more pronounced in children.[1]

Psychotherapies have been relatively infrequently studied in youth with bipolar disorder, although they offer the option of decreased risks relative to medications. Both family-focused and cognitive-behavioral therapy (CBT) approaches are promising, particularly for bipolar depression and relapse prevention, although content must be adjusted for the child's age. Successful treatment of youth with bipolar disorder, as with adults, requires a programmatic approach as described in Chapter 9, including systematic psychopharmacology, appropriate targeted psychotherapies, education and family involvement, mood charting, and good general health measures.

> *Key Point*: Pediatric bipolar disorder cannot simply be assumed to be the same as bipolar disorder in adults. Differences in diagnosis and treatment require somewhat different strategies in order to achieve maximal outcomes.

10.2. Late-Life Bipolar Disorder

Bipolar disorder is less common in late life, due in large part to the younger age of mortality associated with the illness (see Chapter 4). Nonetheless, the prevalence of bipolar disorder in people over age 60 years is up to 0.4%, comprising 10–25% of cases of mood disorders in this age group.[2,3] In older bipolar individuals, manic and psychotic symptoms tend to be less pronounced, so that depressive symptoms predominate even more than in younger ages; otherwise, diagnostic and course-of-illness considerations are similar across the adult age span. Risks from depression and mania related to higher rates of medical illness must be considered, for example, injury from falls during impulsive behavior, and risk of suicide increases with age as well.

In most cases, late-life bipolar disorder is simply a continuation of illness from the typical onset ages of 15–25 years. New-onset bipolar disorder, defined by new-onset mania, becomes less common after age 35 years and is quite uncommon after age 50 years. In this latter group, new-onset mania should be considered a consequence of an underlying medical condition until proven otherwise.[2–4] The more frequent medical causes of new-onset mania in older individuals are listed in Box 10.1, although, again, they are relatively uncommon.[4]

Treatment of bipolar disorder in older adults is complicated by several factors. First, there are few clinical studies in this age group, so that neither efficacy nor tolerability of standard therapies is well defined. Second, late-life bipolar disorder is complicated by significantly higher rates of medical comorbidity that may alter drug disposition and metabolism. Finally, psychotherapies have rarely been studied with particular attention to the needs and concerns of older adults. Nonetheless several guidelines can be followed.[2,3]

With aging, drug metabolism decreases. Consequently, medication doses that are tolerable in midlife become toxic with aging. Therefore, when starting a new medication, begin at one-half to one-third of the standard adult dose and then titrate more slowly, monitoring carefully for tolerability while assessing efficacy. For drugs with relevant serum levels, check these more frequently until a stable therapeutic level is achieved. At the first sign of new symptoms, particularly those suggestive of delirium (e.g., confusion), reevaluate all medications that are being prescribed, even if they have been taken for years. For

---

Box 10.1 Medical Causes of Mania in Late Life

Stroke
  Head trauma
  Brain tumor
  Dementia
  Epilepsy
  CNS infection
  Hemodialysis
  Brain injury after surgery
  Normal pressure hydrocephalus
  Vitamin B12 deficiency

example, a person on lithium 1,200 mg for 20 years with a long-standing serum level of 0.6 meq/L can relatively suddenly develop toxicity with renal function decline after age 65 years. Moreover, some antipsychotics have been associated with sudden death in older adults. Electroconvulsive therapy may be a higher level choice in this age group than in younger individuals as it might be better tolerated and safer. Otherwise, medication choices are largely guided by the same decision processes as in younger adults. Finally, psychotherapies must incorporate the stresses of later life including decreased ability to sleep, declining physical health, and loss of spouse, partners, and friends. In older individuals, following a systematic, deliberate approach as described in Chapter 9 is perhaps even more important than in younger individuals, with a focus on minimizing the number of medications prescribed.

> *Key Point*: Managing bipolar disorder in late life requires increased attention to co-occurring medical problems as well as changes in drug distribution and metabolism.

10.3. Bipolar Disorder and Pregnancy

Managing bipolar disorder during pregnancy is complex. Pregnancy, and especially childbirth, is a high-risk period for relapse in bipolar women. Unfortunately, many bipolar disorder treatments are teratogenic (Table 10.2). Lithium is associated with a three- to eight-fold increased risk of cardiac malformation, namely Ebstein's anomaly, a malformation of tricuspid valve formation leading to cardiac conduction and ejection problems. The antiepileptic medications carbamazepine and divalproex are associated with up to a 20-fold increased risk of neural tube and craniofacial malformations. These malformations occur with first-trimester exposure. Moreover, many benzodiazepines are contraindicated in pregnancy, and antidepressants are typically USFDA class C as well. Risks from other standard treatments are largely undefined. In all cases, very little is known of the long-term neurodevelopmental risks that might result from *in utero* exposure to psychotropic medications. However, untreated mania and depression impart increased risks of miscarriage, premature delivery, and fetal underdevelopment. Consequently,

Table 10.2 Bipolar Disorder Medications in Pregnancy

Medication	USFDA Rating
Lithium	D
Atypical antipsychotics	C
Divalproex	D
Carbamazepine	D
Lamotrigine	C
Oxcarbazepine	C

The FDA classifies drug safety in pregnancy using the following categories: A = controlled studies show no risk; B = no evidence of risk in humans; C = risk cannot be ruled out; D = positive evidence of risk.

simply stopping all treatment in a pregnant woman with bipolar disorder may not be appropriate.

In the case of a planned pregnancy, ideally every attempt should be made to minimize medication exposure to the developing baby. If the woman has a history of relatively mild bipolar illness or was previously able to stop medications without rapid relapse, it might be possible to discontinue medications for the entire pregnancy. Alternatively, since most of the teratogenic risk occurs in the first trimester, it may be preferred to discontinue medications only during that time. Regardless, with either approach, medications should be tapered slowly prior to attempts at pregnancy and contingency plans developed in case of relapse.

In many cases, however, pregnancy is unplanned; in these instances, the goal is still to minimize fetal exposure to potentially dangerous medications, so when possible, they should be discontinued as rapidly as deemed safe. However, as noted, since most of the risk occurs in the first trimester, if the pregnancy is not brought to attention until after that period, discontinuing treatment may no longer be the best choice. Fetal ultrasounds may help guide these decisions. In both unplanned and planned pregnancy, when medications are discontinued, psychotherapy and general health measures should be increased and omega-3 fatty acid therapy might be considered. Electroconvulsive therapy is generally safe during pregnancy and offers an alternative, particular for treatment of acute episodes during the first trimester. Given the high risk of relapse at delivery, standard treatment should generally be reinitiated during the final month of pregnancy. In all cases, care must be coordinated among the pregnant woman, her obstetrician, and her psychiatrist with ongoing assessments and discussion of the relative risks of stopping or remaining on treatment.

> *Key Point*: Managing pregnancy in women with bipolar disorder is complex, requiring careful risk-versus-benefit calculations of whether or not to remain on medications at various stages of the pregnancy. The decisions require well-coordinated assessments and discussions among the pregnant woman, her obstetrician, and her psychiatrist.

10.4. Rapid Cycling

Rapid cycling is defined as four or more distinct affective episodes within a single year. A critical aspect of this definition is that the episodes are *distinct*. Typically, this criterion is defined by a polarity switch (e.g., from mania to depression) or an affective episode recurrence after at least 8 weeks of remission. A relapse, that is, a new full episode, occurring after symptom improvement but before 8 weeks is considered a continuation of the current episode, rather than a new episode. Additionally, mania is often characterized by mood lability, namely, rapid mood changes and fluctuations during the course of the day that can include depressed mood (see Chapter 2). Consequently, mood lability is not "ultrarapid cycling" as it is sometimes mistakenly called. During mixed states, fluctuations among manic and depressive symptoms occur, but

Life events (stress)
    Sleep disruption
    Drug abuse
    Alcohol abuse
    Thyroid disease
    Other medical illness
    Antidepressant use
    Stimulant use
    Treatment nonadherence

represent a single mixed episode rather than "rapid cycling." Mixed and manic episodes, including those with mood lability are managed according to mania treatment algorithms.

When it occurs, rapid cycling is typically a time-limited response to a specific trigger. Common causes of rapid cycling are listed in Box 10.2. The first goal in managing rapid cycling, then, is to identify the underlying precipitant and address it while concurrently maximizing relapse-prevention therapy; that is, increase mood stabilizer doses as tolerated, add a second mood stabilizer, or switch to an alternative drug. While addressing rapid cycling, remember the core treatment principles of systematic drug changes while prescribing three or fewer psychotropic medications if possible. In general, maintenance therapy that prevents *both* mania and depression is preferred; lithium may be less effective in rapid cycling than other choices.

> *Key Point*: Rapid cycling is typically a time-limited state caused by a precipitant; the first response, then, is to manage the precipitant.

10.5. Managing Suicidal Individuals with Bipolar Disorder

Suicide is a tragic and all too common consequence of bipolar disorder. Up to 50% of people with bipolar disorder attempt suicide, and about 15% kill themselves. This rate is 30 times higher than in the general population. Fortunately, with increasing treatment availability and awareness, this rate may now be decreasing; nonetheless, suicide remains a significant concern in the management of bipolar disorder.[5]

There are several steps clinicians can take to help decrease the risk of suicide in people with bipolar disorder. A critical step is to make suicide assessment a routine part of appointments, particularly during periods of high risk. Discussing suicide does not increase the risk of suicide and in fact, this simple intervention likely diminishes the risk. Many individuals are ambivalent about suicide, so talking about these thoughts with an empathic clinician may help the individual move forward to better solutions. Similarly, clinicians can assist family members so that they, too, are comfortable with these discussions and can participate in a nonjudgmental supportive and problem-solving manner.

A second component of managing suicide is to recognize risk factors (Table 10.3).[5] Some of these cannot be modified, but nonetheless provide context for risk assessment. Others can be addressed through changes in treatment or lifestyle. Within these risks are inflection points, such as hospitalization, switch into a mixed state, relapse of drug or alcohol abuse, developing a new major medical illness, or the occurrence of another major life stress (e.g., divorce or loss), that indicate a need for increased vigilance for suicidal behavior. In particular, mixed states and rapid cycling elevate suicide risk by energizing depressed and hopeless individuals. Finally, there are also protective factors that aid assessment and can be enhanced (Table 10.3).

When an individual expresses suicidal thoughts, a careful assessment of acute and chronic risk factors, inflection points, and the presence of protective factors is used to determine whether hospitalization is necessary. If hospitalization is not needed, then developing clear contingency plans during outpatient care for increasing suicidal thoughts will help both the bipolar individual and their family members manage these impulses. Over the long term,

Table 10.3 Suicide Risk and Protective Factors in Bipolar Disorder
Risk Factors
Prior suicide attempts
Family history of suicide
Suicidal ideation
Mixed state
Depression
Hopelessness
Rapid cycling
Drug/Alcohol abuse
Anxiety/Panic attacks
Psychosis
Personality disorder
Early onset illness
Recent loss
Major life stressor
Chronic medical illness
Protective Factors
Supportive family/children at home
Strong religious beliefs
Strong social support
Future orientation
Good coping skills
Ongoing mental health care
Limited access to highly lethal methods of suicide (e.g., guns)
Source: Goodwin and Jamison[5]

with chronic suicidal ideation in particular, treatment must be tailored to assist the bipolar individual in building more protective factors while minimizing risks; therapy can be targeted to manage suicidal impulses and the underlying risk factors by developing alternative adaptive behaviors. Finally, as noted in Chapter 7, lithium decreases suicide risk unlike other treatments; consequently, lithium may be the treatment of choice in suicidal individuals, although because of the risks associated with overdose, it may need to be prescribed in frequent but small amounts for safety. Regardless, suicide remains a complex behavior that is often impulsive and difficult to predict. By approaching the treatment of bipolar disorder comprehensively as described in this book, it is hoped that the risk of this tragic outcome can be ameliorated.

> *Key Point:* Suicide is a significant risk in bipolar disorder; management requires ongoing support of protective factors while compensating for risk factors and acute stressors.

10.6. Managing Comorbidities

As discussed in Chapter 4, bipolar disorder is commonly complicated by co-occurring psychiatric, medical, and substance use disorders. Consequently, most bipolar individuals will require treatment for these other conditions. The vast number of potential combinations exceeds the scope of this book, so only general guidelines are provided here.

10.6.1. Substance Use Disorders

Drug and alcohol abuse occur in more than half of individuals with bipolar disorder. These conditions negatively impact course of illness, so must be addressed as part of the overall treatment of bipolar disorder. Historically, some self-help groups advocated against any medication use in people recovering from drug or alcohol addictions regardless of other conditions; this stance is clearly not reasonable for individuals with bipolar disorder, since mood stabilizers are critical for wellness. Conversely, some psychiatrists advocate for not treating the bipolar disorder until co-occurring substance abuse has remitted. This position is also untenable, as recurrent mood episodes and the associated stresses set up these individuals for addiction relapse and worsening course of bipolar illness. Consequently, both bipolar and substance use disorders must be managed concurrently when they co-occur.

Because there is currently minimal overlap in effective medications for bipolar and substance use disorders, if drugs are used for the latter, these typically will need to be added to an existing effective mood-stabilizing regimen, again, keeping in mind the "three or fewer psychotropic medications" rule of Chapters 7 and 9 and monitoring for negative adverse effects and drug-drug interactions. In contrast, there is overlap in cognitive/behavioral strategies for both conditions that might provide an integrated approach; several research groups are developing specific bipolar and substance use disorders integrated therapy manuals (see Weiss and Connery[6] as an example).

Regardless, standard approaches to drug and alcohol abuse should be initiated as soon as possible in bipolar individuals with these conditions. Research also suggests that the year after a first hospitalization for mania is a very high risk time for the onset of drug and alcohol use, so that preventative intervention during this period is warranted.

> Key Point: The best overall approach for managing co-occurring bipolar and substance use disorders is to aggressively identify the best treatment regimen possible for bipolar illness while concurrently initiating aggressive therapies for the substance use disorder. When possible, integrated treatment for both conditions is preferable.

10.6.2. Co-occurring Psychiatric Conditions

In addition to substance use disorders, other psychiatric conditions commonly co-occur in bipolar disorder (Chapter 4). Although each combination and individual present unique challenges, the general approach toward managing these situations proceeds as follows.

The top priority is to maximize mood stabilization for the bipolar illness, since bipolar disorder is typically the more disabling condition. Additionally, interventions for other psychiatric illnesses (e.g., OCD) may require treatments (e.g., antidepressants) that can destabilize bipolar disorder if it is not appropriately managed first. Moreover, some apparent comorbidity (e.g., anxiety symptoms) may resolve with improvement in the primary bipolar illness. The exception to this rule is if the second condition is interfering with obtaining mood stabilization, then it should be concurrently managed using interventions that do not disrupt treatment for bipolar disorder. For example, an individual with both bipolar and borderline personality disorders might not be able to participate in treatment for bipolar disorder without initiating dialectical behavioral therapy for the personality disorder, in order to improve behavioral control and treatment adherence.

Once mood stabilization is established, then aggressive management of the second condition ensues. Ideally, when possible, it is best to use therapies that are effective for both conditions, toward the general goal of minimizing polypharmacy and eliminating multiple and potentially competing psychotherapies. Carefully crafted psychotherapy is often a good alternative; for example, a well-designed CBT can assist with bipolar depression and provide primary treatment of co-occurring OCD. Charting symptoms of both conditions to systematically identify effective interventions becomes critical in these complex situations. Again, the general principles of programmatic treatment described in Chapter 9 apply, with expansion to include the second condition.

> Key Point: The best overall approach for managing co-occurring bipolar and other psychiatric disorder is to first stabilize the bipolar illness and then manage the secondary condition, with an eye toward integrated treatments when possible.

10.6.3. Co-occurring Medical Illnesses

Also as described in Chapter 4, individuals with bipolar disorder suffer from higher rates than the general population of many medical conditions such as diabetes, migraine, and cardiovascular disease.[4] There are two primary challenges when managing medical comorbidities in bipolar disorder. First, studies have shown that people with mental illness receive substandard medical care in the community as compared with people without mental illness. Although the specific reasons for this bias are not clear, it is likely that primary and specialist medical providers attribute symptoms of medical illness to the psychiatric condition, thereby discounting them. A second challenge is that primary care providers are often unfamiliar or uncomfortable with psychotropic medications, so may either be reluctant to start standard medical therapies or are unaware of potential drug-drug interactions that negatively impact treatment of bipolar disorder. For example, a simple recommendation of using over-the-counter ibuprofen can lead to lithium toxicity as the former inhibits renal clearance of the latter.

To address these problems, clinicians managing bipolar disorder must serve as advocates for affected individuals within the medical community. Psychiatrists often provide some primary medical care by screening for medical illnesses in order to facilitate treatment referrals. They can also work closely with other physicians to minimize polypharmacy and guard against potentially dangerous drug combinations. Nonpsychiatrists can help their bipolar clients by identifying and establishing referral relationships with medical providers who do not stigmatize people with mental illness and take their physical complaints seriously. In both cases, identifying primary and specialty medical providers who work collaboratively with mental health clinicians offers the best opportunity for people with bipolar disorder to receive optimal medical treatment. Bipolar individuals can facilitate their care by being diligent in seeking treatment for medical symptoms and by working within the local bipolar community to identify the best primary and specialist care providers who work with people with mental illnesses.

> *Key Point*: Managing medical illness in bipolar disorder typically requires active advocacy by mental health providers on behalf of bipolar individuals.

References

1. Geller B, DelBello MP, eds. *Treatment of Bipolar Disorder in Children and Adolescents*. New York: Guilford Press, 2008.

2. Aziz R, Lorberg B, Tampi RR. Treatments for late-life bipolar disorder. Am J Geriatric Pharmacotherapy 2006; 4:347–364.

3. Sajatovic M, Blow FC. *Bipolar Disorder in Later Life*. Baltimore, MD: Johns Hopkins University Press, 2007.

4. Sax KW, Strakowski SM. The co-occurrence of bipolar disorder with medical illness. In: Tohen M, ed., *Comorbidity in Affective Disorders.* New York: Dekker, 1999.

5. Goodwin FK, Jamison KR. Chapter 25: Clinical management of suicide risk. *Manic-Depressive Illness: Bipolar Disorders and Recurrent Depression.* New York: Oxford University Press, 2007.

6. Weiss RD, Connery HS. *Integrated Group Therapy for Bipolar Disorder and Substance Abuse.* New York: Guilford Press, 2011.

Appendix

Example Mood Chart

Day Measurement	1	2	3	4	5	6	7	8	9	10	11	12	13	14	15	16	17	18	19	20	21	22	23	24	25	26	27	28	29	30	31
Medications:																															
Lithium 900 mg	X	X	X	X	X	X				X	X	X	X	X	X	X	X	X	X	X	X	X	X	X	X	X	X	X	X	X	X
Lamotrigine 300 mg																							X	X	X	X	X	X	X	X	X
Alcohol use, glasses	0	1	1	2	1	5	3	6	4	6	4	3	5	5	1	0	0	0	0	0	0	0	1	0	0	1	0	0	0	0	0
Sleep, hours	7	8	7	8	7	4	5	4	3	5	2	2	6	9	9	11	12	12	12	10	10	10	9	8	8	7	6	7	7	7	7
Mood:																															
Severe mania																															
Moderate mania									X	X																					
Mild mania								X			X	X	X	X	X																
Feeling well	X	X	X	X	X	X	X									X	X	X													
Mild depression																											X	X		X	X
Moderate depression																			X	X	X	X	X	X	X	X			X		
Severe depression																															

Example of a mood chart identifying possible items to be measured. In this example individual, discontinuing lithium (day 7) is associated with increased manic symptoms and increased alcohol use, followed by cycling into depression (day 16). Lamotrigine is added on day 23 to address these symptoms. Note changes in sleep associated with mood switches. The changes here are exaggerated for illustration purposes only and should not be viewed necessarily as a typical course or treatment response.

This design is loosely based on the "Personal Calendar" available from the Depression and Bipolar Support Alliance (DBSA). The DBSA sells at a nominal cost a more detailed, 6-month calendar/mood chart that is strongly recommended for any practice in which people with mood disorders receive care. DBSA can be contacted on their web site—www.DBSAlliance.org—or at DBSA, 730 N. Franklin Street, Suite 501, Chicago, IL 60610-7224. (800) 826-3632.

Month: July

Index

Page numbers followed by "b", "f", and "t" indicate boxes, figures, and tables.